Praise for

THE HEALTH HABIT

"Elizabeth Rider has cracked the lifestyle and diet code in a way that will work for anyone, including you! I've worked with Elizabeth for years—she is the real deal. Every woman should get this book."

— CHRISTIANE NORTHRUP, M.D.

New York Times best-selling author of *Women's Bodies, Women's Wisdom* and *Goddesses Never Age*

"Elizabeth has written the ultimate guide to holistic health! *The Health Habit* not only demystifies nutrition, but it also offers up practical and inspiring guidance on every element of well-being."

— GABRIELLE BERNSTEIN

#1 *New York Times* best-selling author of *The Universe Has Your Back*

"*The Health Habit* is a brilliant book for any woman seeking better health without shame or guilt. Elizabeth delivers a clear, compassionate, and actionable plan that will serve you for life."

— MARIE FORLEO

star of MarieTV, entrepreneur, and philanthropist and author of *Everything Is Figureoutable*

"*The Health Habit* is a must-read for anyone looking to better their health. Elizabeth is the queen of mastering simple, practical, and sustainable healthy habits that last."

— JAMES COLQUHOUN

filmmaker of *Food Matters*, *Hungry for Change*, and *Transcendence*; founder of FMTV; and author of *Hungry for Change*

"*The Health Habit* is the best healthy eating and lifestyle book I've read in a long time! The simplicity of the steps and flexibility of this approach will help anyone move toward healthier habits in a realistic manner to create lasting results. This book is now at the top of my list of recommendations to set people on the road to better nutrition and health."

— SUE WARD, M.S., CNS,

director of Nutrition and Education, Sanoviv Medical Institute, and author of *Cruising for Fitness or Finish Lines*

THE
HEALTH HABIT

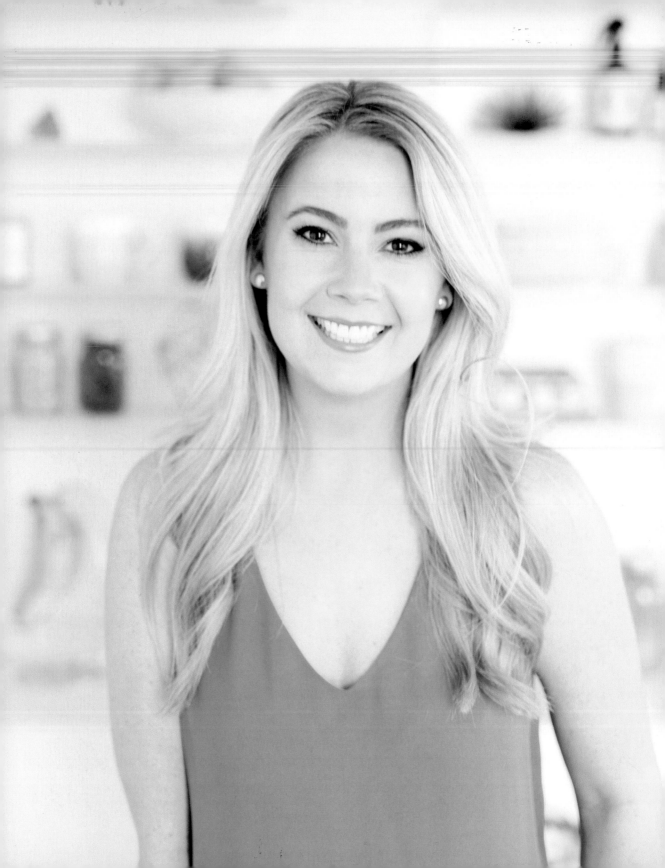

THE
HEALTH HABIT

7 EASY STEPS to Reach Your Goals and Dramatically Improve Your Life

ELIZABETH RIDER

HAY HOUSE, INC.

Carlsbad, California • New York City
London • Sydney • New Delhi

Published in the United States by: Hay House, Inc.: www
.hayhouse.com® • *Published in Australia by:* Hay House
Australia Pty. Ltd.: www.hayhouse.com.au • *Published in the
United Kingdom by:* Hay House UK, Ltd.: www.hayhouse.co.uk •
Published in India by: Hay House Publishers India: www
.hayhouse.co.in

Cover and book design: Shubhani Sarkar, sarkardesignstudio.com
Cover photo: D'Arcy Benincosa, darcybenincosa.com
Interior photos: Samantha Lord, orangephotographie.com and
      Elizabeth Rider, elizabethrider.com
Indexer: J S Editorial, LLC

Library of Congress Cataloging-in-Publication Data
Names: Rider, Elizabeth, author.
Title: The health habit : 7 easy steps to reach your goals and
   dramatically improve your life / Elizabeth Rider.
Description: Carlsbad, California : Hay House Inc., 2019.
Identifiers: LCCN 2019014140| ISBN 9781401956981 (hardback) |
   ISBN 9781401956998 (e-book) | ISBN 9781401958435
   (audiobook)
Subjects: LCSH: Health behavior. | Nutrition. | Weight loss. | Gluten-
   free diet--Recipes. | Milk-free diet--Recipes. | BISAC: HEALTH &
   FITNESS / Nutrition. | HEALTH & FITNESS / Healthy Living. |
   HEALTH & FITNESS / Weight Loss.
Classification: LCC RA776.9 .R54 2019 | DDC 613.2--dc23 LC
   record available at https://lccn.loc.gov/2019014140

Hardcover ISBN: 978-1-4019-5698-1
e-book ISBN: 978-1-4019-5699-8
Audiobook ISBN: 978-1-4019-5843-5

10 9 8 7 6 5 4 3 2 1

1st edition, August 2019
Printed in the United States of America

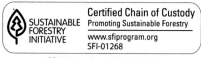

Certified Chain of Custody
Promoting Sustainable Forestry
www.sfiprogram.org
SFI-01268

SFI label applies to the text stock

This book is dedicated to you, dear reader.
May your Health Habit bring you a higher level
of well-being and more joy to your daily life.
You deserve it.

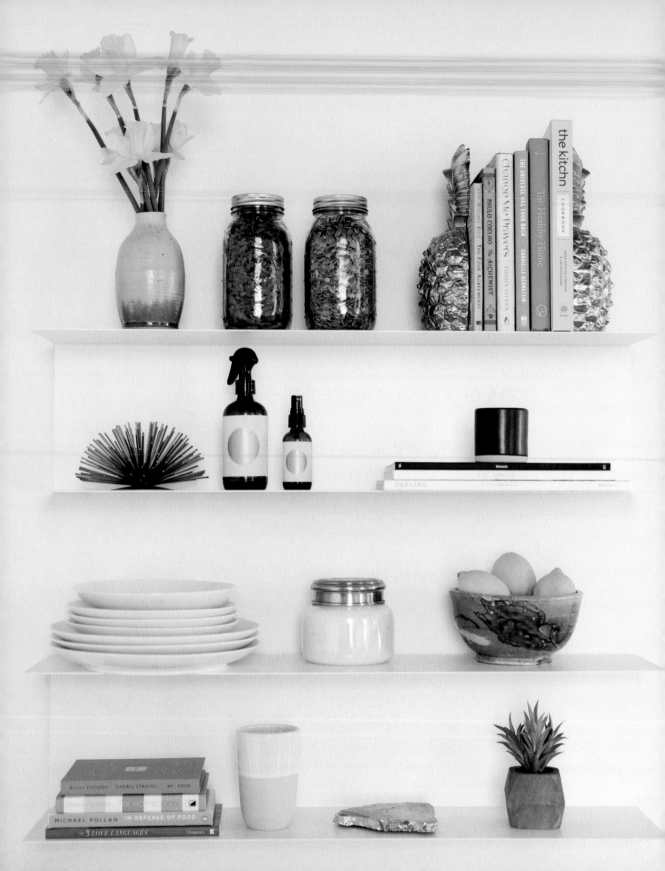

CONTENTS

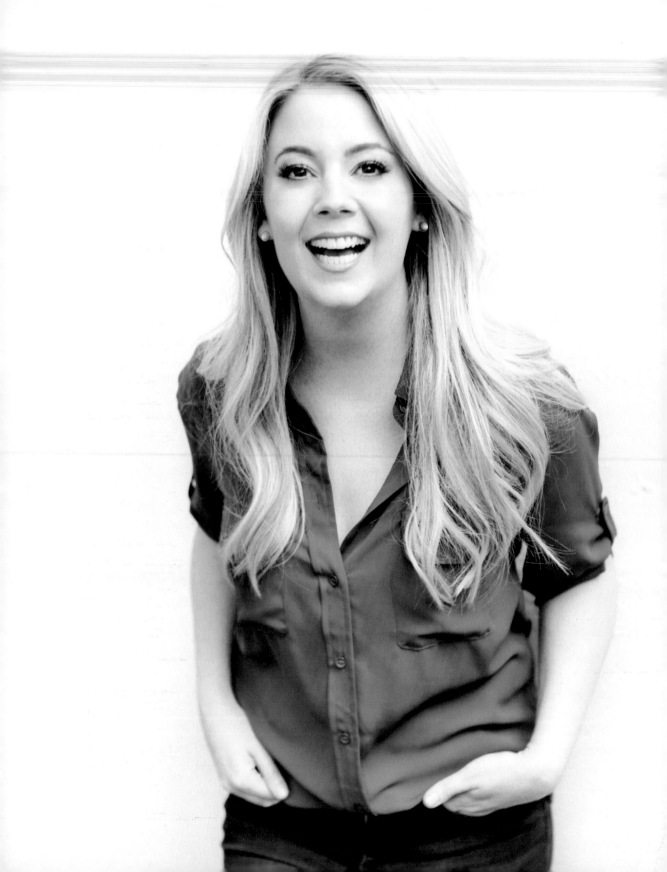

How Healthy Habits Became My Life

If you're like me and want to be healthy without giving up everything you love—and not feel guilty for "messing up"—then this book is for you. Before I tell you my story, I want you to know that I don't expect it to be yours.

This book is designed to meet you where you are, whether you have thyroid problems similar to mine, or you're prediabetic, suffering from an autoimmune disease, looking to lose weight, hoping to lift some brain fog, or simply in the market for tips to improve an already healthy lifestyle. The steps in this book are here to help you jump out of bed on Monday mornings regardless of where you start. In case we've never met before, let me back up a little.

Hi! I'm Elizabeth. It's so nice to meet you. I'm a health coach, nutritionist, recipe blogger, and host of the cooking show *Elizabeth Eats* on FMTV. I grew up in the biggest town in Montana (80,000 people strong), where I lived in a quaint little postwar house with my mom, dad, and two older sisters. We didn't have loads of money, but our home was full of love (and fighting teenage girls from 1994 to 1998). I was a cheerleader (don't judge me) and took dance lessons every week for 18 years. Overall I was a pretty average healthy, happy-go-lucky kind of kid. Until I wasn't.

MY OWN HEALTH STRUGGLES

It started in my early teen years with what seemed to be strep throat every month, followed by antibiotic round after antibiotic round. The doctor decided it was best to take my tonsils out when I was 15, and for years I never fully felt like I recovered from the surgery.

As luck would have it, I got mononucleosis the next year—and not even from kissing (because I was such a prude), which felt even lamer to teenage me. If I had to get sick, I wanted a cool story about it. I contracted mono most likely from sharing sugary drinks with my fellow cheer friends at football games.

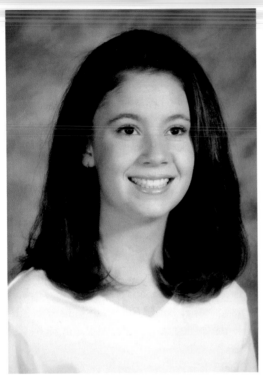

Age 15, right after having my tonsils out

But how I contracted mono doesn't really matter, what's important is I was so sick I missed almost an entire semester of my junior year of high school. And although I started to recover slowly but surely, I did not regain full steam.

The next year, climbing the school stairs a week before graduation, I suddenly had to sit down. I was winded—a strange phenomenon for a teen who was a dancer her entire life. A friend walked me to the nurse's office, and I ended up at the doctor that day. A blood panel revealed thyroid levels so low, I needed to get on medication the very same night.

Over the next 10 or so years, I popped that thyroid medication every morning and didn't think much of it. Except that once again I

didn't ever feel 100 percent better. Improved, sure. But something always felt off. Between bottomed-out energy levels and a few pounds I just couldn't seem to shake, I lived my way into my 30s figuring I'd just have to accept that for some reason my thyroid quit working. Years later, after committing to figuring out my health, I discovered the idea of reactivation of the Epstein-Barr virus (EBV).

After a lot of confusing testing, hours upon hours of reading and researching other people's stories, and absorbing all the information I could get my hands on, I asked my naturopath for an EBV test: It came back with sky-high antibodies of a recent infection. This was a huge surprise, because my diagnosis with mono was 15 years earlier.

Turns out that my low thyroid and constantly feeling tired all these years could possibly be attributed back to the first bout of mono and a chronic case of EBV. (If you want to read more about my EBV diagnosis, testing, and treatment, you can find all of that on my website, elizabethrider.com.)

I had to take my health into my own hands, and that's what this book is here to teach you. It doesn't matter whether you suspect your diagnosis may be the same as mine, struggle with a similar story, or just simply feel defeated despite knowing how to live healthfully but not following through.

The action steps for building a healthy lifestyle that you'll find in this book will help you support your best health through positive changes that will serve you forever. Here, you'll learn how to create healthy habits that work for you. And I don't mean you'll be living a sterile, indulgent-free life. I mean that you will both see results and look forward to continuing these new healthy habits.

Because while you can get results from just about any health program out there, if you don't love your daily life, sticking with it may feel like torture. The road to vibrant health should feel expansive, not restrictive.

WHAT I'VE DISCOVERED

After years of feeling run down and struggling with my own healthy lifestyle, what I do know is this: When I started looking at my health from a full daily lifestyle perspective—where all areas, not just food, mattered—everything changed. I also know that while I can stick to any diet under the sun for a period of time, none of them felt sustainable for the long haul.

I turned to nutrition, first, and slowly but surely began experimenting. I became a certified health coach and immersed myself in dozens of different healing modalities from around the world. I studied more than 100 different dietary theories, committed myself in emotional healing techniques, completed my Pilates and yoga teacher trainings, and attended healing retreats all over the world to learn more about concepts like Ayurveda (India's ancient system of medicine) and all-natural therapies that have dramatic positive effects on the body.

I completed the Cornell University Plant-Based Nutrition Program and integrated those teachings with my full-circle approach. I

———

Your health is your greatest asset.

———

completed all three levels of Sanoviv Medical Institute's Nutrition Advisor program to understand what cutting-edge approaches are available. (Spoiler alert: Food really is medicine.)

I learned what it meant to be healthy and well from all angles, and how undeniably important our emotional, spiritual, and environmental health are to preventing manifestation of disease in the body. I learned that eating real food helps, and most processed food delivers four seconds of pleasure for four hours of feeling like crap. That cutting out harmful chemicals from beauty and home products was easier than I thought, and how small lifestyle tweaks here and there made all the difference in my health.

DOES A HEALTHY LIFESTYLE EVEN MATTER?

In case you need a little kick in the tush to make an effort to live a healthier lifestyle, I want to remind you that you provide a tremendous amount of value to the world and people around you. Even if you don't feel it at this moment, no one is born by accident.

You're here to positively affect the people and world around you, be it your immediate family, a small group of kids you volunteer with, the team you lead at work, one patient in a therapy session, or the thousands whom you affect as an entrepreneur. Impacting the world and people around you becomes increasingly difficult if you don't feel your best.

Your health is your greatest asset. It's not

your house, that 401k you've worked so hard to build, your savings, or your job. If you have your health, you can do anything. Without your health, your time, energy, and resources are consumed with not feeling well.

When you have your health, your time is opened up to do the great work you are here to do. Your people need you, and the world needs you. If that's not enough, here are three more reasons why all of this matters:

Reason #1:
The Rise of "Lifestyle Diseases"

Autoimmune disease diagnosis is on the rise at staggering rates, and we know that most autoimmune disease begins in the digestive tract (aka gut). And guess where all your food goes? In case you skipped your middle-school health class, the answer is your gut.

The good news is that the cells lining the inside of the gut turn over every three to seven days, so you *can* heal the lining of your gut and improve your health with food and lifestyle changes.

Chronic conditions such as heart disease, type 2 diabetes, hypertension, obesity, and certain types of cancer are on the rise at alarming rates all around the world. These diseases are known as "lifestyle diseases" because they are largely preventable by means of diet and habit changes.

The number-one cause of death in the United States (and most developed countries) is heart disease. A recent study by the U.S. Centers for Disease Control and Prevention found that more than 50 percent of deaths from coronary artery disease (a type of heart disease) can be attributed to preventable factors such as eating unhealthy foods, poor physical activity, or heavy consumption of alcohol.[1]

Prevention of lifestyle-related disease starts with establishing healthy habits at home and in your kitchen.

Reason #2:
The Hidden Face of Aging

You *can* slow the aging process. And I'm not talking about chasing a version of unattainable Hollywood youth.

Now that you know that the world needs you—there will never be another you—I want you to realize that you deserve to feel good on a daily basis. You have two ages: your chronological age and your biological age. Your chronological age is just a number on your driver's license and passport. In my opinion, the more important of the two is your biological age—that is, the age of your cells.

The phenom that is your body is made of more than 50 trillion cells. To put that in perspective, one million seconds is about eleven and a half days. One billion seconds is about 31 years! And a trillion seconds? That's 300 centuries ago, before there was even a written history. I share these numbers to remind you of how miraculous it is that you're even alive.

Back to how we measure our age. On the outside, we may judge age by the look of our skin. But that's just the beginning.

More important than those face lines you love and hate is the biological age of the inside of your body. Giving your cells the antiaging power of a healthy lifestyle will do far more than any single antiaging cream on the market, and—more important—it will give you a higher quality of life for a longer period of time.

Let's get science-y for a moment: Advanced glycation end products (AGEs) can form in the body when sugars bind to some of our DNA, proteins, and lipids (fats). As my friend and biochemist Dr. Libby Weaver explains, this process can cause cells and tissues to not work properly, resulting in aging or, in some cases, disease.[2]

You have full control over how you feed your 50 trillion cells, and giving them what they need to thrive starts with daily Health Habits. Not a 10-day cleanse or short-term exercise plan. It's your day in and day out healthy habits over time that count.

You deserve to feel good in your own skin. What that means is different for everyone. While it's important not to chase photoshopped beauty that we all know isn't real, it's completely normal, and biologically ingrained, to want to feel good.

And while you know that looking like an airbrushed model shot from a perfect angle is unattainable, wanting to have the energy to play with your kids and feel confident in your clothes is your birthright.

One of the most common phrases I hear from my clients is, "I know life isn't all about weight, but I just know I feel better at a certain weight. Is that vain?" The answer to that question is no. I'll say it again: *You are worthy of feeling good in your own skin.* You deserve it and you're worth it.

It's been observed that people weigh more today than they did 20 or 30 years ago even though they are not necessarily consuming more food or exercising less.[3] Think about that: a person is predicted to weigh more today than

What You'll Find in This Book:

- Action steps to create a healthy lifestyle you love.

- Relatable advice from real-life experiences. (I love food, too, and I'm not here to take away everything you like to eat and resign you to an eternity of plain chicken breast and steamed broccoli.)

- The truth about diets, nutrition, and health. Spoiler alert: It isn't always black and white.

- Exercises to help you gain the self-awareness you need to make positive lifestyle changes.

- Encouragement to try different things. In order to create positive change, you'll have to be willing to change some of your thinking.

- Recommendations that are reasonable for your time and budget. If your new habits don't fit your reality, you'll end up right back where you started.

in the late 1980s even while eating the same amount of food (even adjusted for the ratios of protein, fats, and carbohydrates consumed) and exercising the same amount.

But why? While this observation has been confirmed by scientific study, the causes are mostly still hypothetical. Many, myself included, suggest that lab-created food, toxins

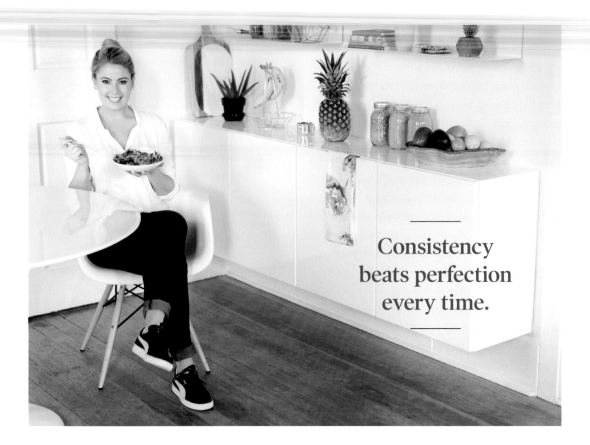

Consistency
beats perfection
every time.

in beauty products and the environment, excessive stress, low-quality sleep, and hormonal imbalances caused by said stress and toxins are all contributing factors.

Reason #3: Quality of Life

Remember, you are meant to feel good. The notion that it's normal to not feel well as you age—whether you're in your 20s or 60s—is a myth. The phrase "We live too short and we die too long" has never been more true. There's no proof that feeling unwell is a necessary part of life.

Not feeling well is an indication that something is off. Your body is a fine piece of machinery that will wear and tear with age, and small cracks and squeaks are common. But feeling unwell for long periods of time is not how you are meant to live, at any age.

Instead of a prescribed diet, this book is all about building daily habits that will turn into a healthy lifestyle you'll actually look forward to living. There are loads of books out there about how we age, individual dietary theories, and the science behind the body. But few give guidance on how to implement healthy living on a day-to-day basis.

Most books focus on one specific diet or one step of the process. It's not that these books aren't useful—I own many of them—it's that reading about theory doesn't teach you how to set up your life so that healthy living is something you want to embrace.

This book focuses on action, not just theory. I'll reference the science and theory when needed, but we're going to focus on building a life that makes the action feel exciting. And for my fact-finder friends out there, you can take comfort in knowing that the information in this book is rooted in science and has been fact-checked from top to bottom.

HOW TO GET THE MOST OUT OF THIS BOOK

You're not in trouble or being punished. No shame allowed for past decisions. In fact, releasing guilt, shame, and fear is a big part of healing and achieving your highest level of well-being. You're in the here and now, so consider today day one.

I ask that you read these pages with an open mind, and don't assume *I already know that*. Try to stop your inner critic from telling you that something won't work because you're different, or that your goals for healthy living will never happen because you've tried before and it didn't work. These steps work in harmony together. Trust me.

Don't slip into overwhelm. You don't have to do every single thing in this book at once, or even at all. Take what serves you and leave the rest. But take a lot. For real! This stuff works.

That said, read the whole book. While you don't have to take action in the order that these chapters are laid out here, they all intersect at some point. So read all the chapters and then follow the 28-Day Kick-Start Plan in Chapter 9 to get the most benefit from these teachings.

Let go of perfectionism. You'll learn this as we go, and it's worth mentioning here, too: Consistency beats perfection every time because perfection doesn't exist. No person is perfect. I'm going to teach you how to create a lifestyle that helps you keep up with your habits, not one that tells you to be perfect every minute of life. The purpose of this book is to help you create a consistency in your wellness habits and an environment that allows you to thrive.

Now, I've got some good news and some bad news. I'll give you the bad news first because I like to end on a high note (and I don't want you to stop reading this book). The bad news: If you're looking for a black-and-white checklist of exactly what to do to become your healthiest self, you're going to be disappointed. That kind of list doesn't exist.

Trust me, if I could snap my fingers and give the surefire bullet points to lead you to health, I would. But that's not how it works. Every experience you've ever had in life has brought you to where you are now, so only you have the power to untangle the habits that no longer serve you.

The good news: Once you decide to make positive changes in one area of your life, it's easier to make positive changes in other areas, too. We're going to do it together, one step at a time.

The even better news: I designed a 28-Day Kick-Start Plan and community to get you going, keep you motivated, and help you connect with like-minded women from around the world.

Let's get started!

Part I

SECRETS OF HEALTHIER FOOD HABITS

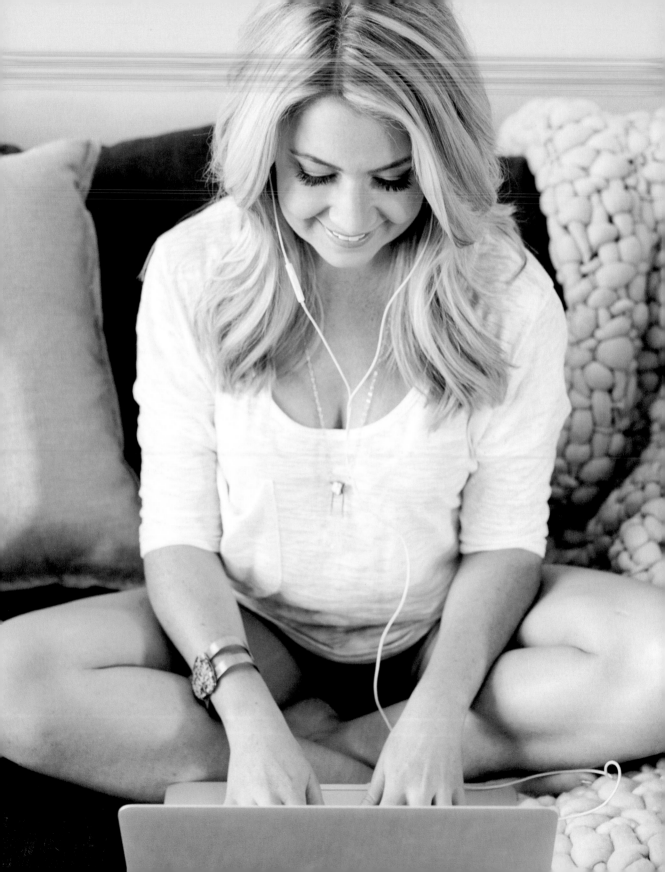

CHAPTER 1

Set Your Goals Straight

*There's a right way—and a wrong way—
to set health goals you can achieve.*

After spending way too long living a healthy lifestyle but not enjoying my life, I've now found a better way. And I'm here to share it with you. You picked up this book because, like me, you want to feel healthy and, like me, you don't want to have to go on another diet, starvation cleanse, or extreme detox to make it happen.

Most likely you know you could feel better, although you just can't put your finger on what's holding you back. Or, you have an inkling of what the problem is, but you don't know what steps to take first. Don't worry, dear reader, I've got you. I was there not too long ago, and after going through the steps outlined in this book, I feel better than ever. At 36, I can honestly say I feel healthier than I felt at 26. And 46 and beyond definitely doesn't scare me. Because I know I can keep feeling healthy and my future is something I look forward to. Together, you and I are going to work on taking action to create healthier habits in all parts of your life.

Research shows that when you improve habits in one area of your life, it's easier to build better habits in other places, too. It all always comes full circle to create your highest (or lowest) level of well-being possible. I've made it my life's mission to share what I've learned on my own path to healing, so you can create the life and health you know you deserve.

Dramatic change does not have to be traumatic. Shocking, I know! Quick-fix media headlines and diet dogma have made us believe that in order to become the healthiest versions of ourselves possible, we have to live in flavorless boxes of perfection. As if there's only one way to be healthy, and it's called the diet highway where if we slip up even once it was all for naught.

Most, if not all, of those dogmatic ways of thinking are false. They've led you astray. While you do have to make the effort—you can't just make one small change and then quit—transforming yourself into a healthy, feel-good-in-your-own-skin, status-quo can't-keep-up-with-her kind of woman doesn't have to mean giving up everything you enjoy and resigning yourself to a life of counting calories or weighing your food.

THE F-WORD WILL SET YOU FREE

I love the F-word, but it might not be the one you're thinking.

In my own personal experience, and from observing the thousands of women who have completed my online programs, I believe that working toward the feeling of *freedom*—in all areas of life—is what leads to the highest levels of well-being. Freedom from the guilt we feel around food choices, freedom from negative self-talk, and freedom from knowing we can feel better but not understanding how to make it happen.

And I know this for sure: You have to create your own freedom. No one else—not your husband, wife, parents, girlfriend, or doctor—can do it for you. Your freedom is your responsibility, and it's absolutely attainable. You just need a plan. (Hint: It's in this book.)

Women are fiercely strong creatures. When we want something, we can commit and become unstoppable. Finish your master's degree while pregnant and working full-time? Not a problem. Train for a marathon while leading a team of executives through a $500 million project, all while taking care of your mother every night? Yep! Done.

Raise four kids while maintaining a home, leading a church group, and volunteering at your kids' school every day? Not a problem. We can dig our nails onto the cliff and hold on for dear life, all while frosting the bake sale cookies, delivering the multimedia report of

> Dramatic change does not have to be traumatic.

the century, and proving our parents wrong (a traveling food blogger *can* make a living, after all). So why does something as seemingly simple as making healthy choices feel so hard? I've sat on this question for years, until it hit me: Because most healthy choices feel like a loss of freedom. But it doesn't have to be that way.

Any lifestyle habits you cultivate or changes you choose to implement should all work toward helping you feel *more* free, never restricted. Expansive, not small.

Choosing to be healthy should make you free from the guilt, shame, and negative chatter that usually comes along with going on a diet or "lifestyle" plan. Because negative emotions can be just as bad for you as the crappy food you're drawn to.

Now, that's not a get-out-of-jail-free card when it comes to how you eat. You still have to care, and you still have to eat real food. You still have to actively try to feel good and put in the effort . . . but that effort doesn't have to feel so damn hard.

As such, this is not a diet book. I'm not going to ask you to eat kale every day for the rest of your life if you're just not that into it.

But I *am* going to ask you to put in the feel-good kind of effort it will take to make some positive changes, because these shifts will dramatically improve your well-being. It's the kind of effort you don't hesitate to spend researching the best restaurants to visit on your next vacation, caring for your loved ones, or showing your boss what an overachieving woman you are.

Now it's time to concentrate on feeling better. It's time to prioritize you.

ESTABLISHING YOUR HEALTH HABIT

Your Health Habit is unique to you. Not a diet, your Health Habit is a skill, or a set of skills, that allows you to make the best choices that serve you most.

There isn't one magic health bullet that works for everyone. Your Health Habit comprises the daily actions that allow you to be the best version of yourself, physically, mentally, and emotionally. Instead of prescribing a list of exactly what to do each day, I'm going to teach you the skill of making the best choices that benefit your overall health. In order to make better choices throughout the day, you have to enjoy your habits. Where you're from and where you currently live, your cultural background, current life conditions, and all of your life experience up until now affects that state of your habits. Not only that, your values and beliefs influence what you enjoy.

To make positive shifts in your habits, first you need to understand that there are three parts to all habits:

1. the cue (aka trigger)

2. the action (aka routine)

3. the reward (aka the benefit)

Researchers at the Massachusetts Institute of Technology have identified the cycle of those three parts as the habit loop. What you think of as the habit is generally the middle part—the action or routine—like putting sugar in your coffee or eating ice cream after dinner every night.

The cue or trigger can be physical (low blood sugar or feeling hungry) or emotional (frustration, boredom, or simply seeking pleasure). The reward generally alleviates the problem that cued it in the first place. If hunger (the cue) causes you to eat ice cream at 8 each night (the action) and that leads to feeling full for a while (the reward), it's possible to just change the action (choose something healthier to satisfy your hunger).

Hunger is a cue that can pretty easily be alleviated by a healthier action. Emotional cues or triggers like frustration at work, boredom in your relationship, or feeling blue from a health condition can take more work to identify, but they can absolutely be shifted as well.

Only you can identify the habit loops you've created. That's why we'll talk about self-awareness often as you build your new Health Habit. The more aware you are of your cues and triggers, and what you're seeking in the reward, the easier it will be to shift your habits.

It's not just about replacing the ice cream with a bag of carrots—you can do that for a week, but it usually won't last because the perceived reward isn't the same. It's about having the self-awareness to understand what's driving your habits in order to shift them.

Sometimes it's as simple as changing the cue, which is why we talk about keeping home-cooked food around and detoxing your home environment. Sometimes it's about finding an enjoyable replacement for the routine/action part of the habit, and sometimes it's about identifying the emotional or physical reward you are after, which can take a little bit of work but is a skill that will serve you for life.

As I mentioned before, this book is action-oriented and aims to help you enjoy your life more, not less. Pretty soon, your Health Habit will be on autopilot and you'll have the skills you need to make positive changes as needed.

THERE'S A RIGHT WAY—
AND A WRONG WAY—
TO SET YOUR GOALS

The first step in creating healthy habits that last for life is to rethink how you set your health goals. I can't think of a single instance in which a client who was having a hard time meeting a goal had set her goal correctly in the first place. This is the reason most people don't hit their goals, and it is simple to fix. There are three progressive parts to setting a goal:

1. Identify the desired feeling

2. Outline daily actionable steps

3. Name the desired outcome

These are taught in the context of good business principles but often aren't translated to health or habits at home—until now! Most people miss thinking through parts one and two, and incorrectly identify number three as the goal—then they fail miserably at trying to achieve it. Even worse, the stress and negative self-talk contribute to the downward spiral of self-sabotage and resistance.

Identifying step one, what you truly desire, is the foundation of any action you take in life. Ultimately, even self-sabotage is a form of taking action on what we desire, as our negative self-talk can lead to the subconscious desire to fail.

To set a foundation and learn how to meet your goals, the very first step is determining what you desire. The how-tos of any process aren't going to do you any good if you don't get this down first. (Hint: Losing 10 pounds is not a desire or a goal. It's an outcome.)

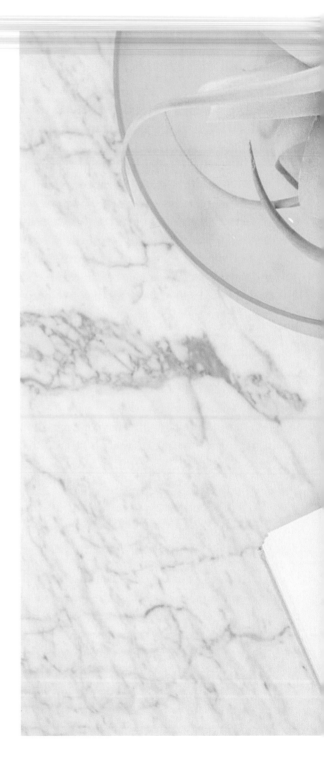

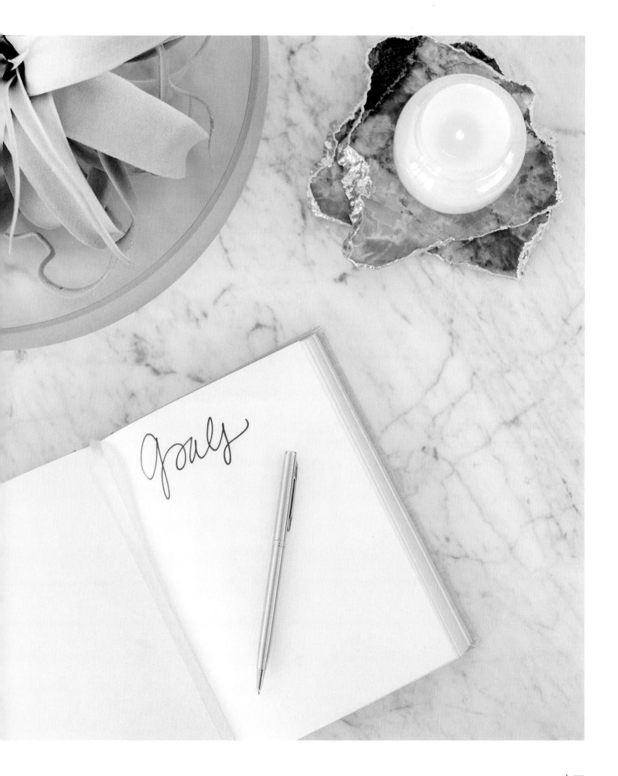

THE FOUR REASONS YOU'RE NOT MEETING YOUR GOALS

Mistake #1:
Confusing the outcome for the goal.

You probably have an outcome in mind, but an outcome isn't a goal. Everyone does this.

Important practical life skills—such as the right way to set goals, negotiating a raise at work, and budgeting for rent, utilities, and groceries—are not usually taught in school or at home. Some of us have some catching up to do and that's okay. Let's start with goals. Losing 10 pounds, fitting into your skinny jeans, or feeling confident in your clothes are not goals. The first two are outcomes and the third is a desire. Goals are the daily actionable habits in between that get you there. Hitting 10,000 steps per day, sticking to a reasonable intermittent fasting window without starving yourself (don't fret, I'll cover this later), eating salmon on Sunday nights, and consuming only low-glycemic foods at breakfast are all daily actionable goals.

Mistake #2:
Misunderstanding the feeling you desire.

Desire is the unseen fire that fuels your daily habits. If you lack motivation to stick to your goals, there's a disconnect between what you desire and the actions that you set for yourself. If your desired outcome is to lose 20 pounds but you're not even the least bit interested in putting better food in your mouth, it's because you know deep down that losing 20 pounds isn't going to change you as a person (and, you're right, it won't). It might be that you don't really desire to be thin, but you desire to

have the feelings that you associate with being thinner. What goes along with being at the weight you want to achieve? Could it be feeling more confident in your clothes? Perhaps to feel more energetic and thus able to spend more time with the people you love?

Your desire can't be just, "I want to be thinner." There's not enough fuel in that statement to motivate you to make it happen. Author Danielle LaPorte literally put desires on the map in her book *The Desire Map,* in which she lists dozens of potential core desired feelings you may wish to achieve. Some of my favorites are:

abundant	healthy (obvi!)
accomplished	holy
adventurous	joyous
alive	natural
authentic	open-hearted
balanced	passionate
brave	powerful
brilliant	prosperous
celebratory	purposeful
centered	regal
cherished	romantic
confident	seen
delighted	sensual
desired	sexy
divine	sincere
elegant	spirited
energized	supported
fabulous	thankful
feminine	vibrant
generous	warm
healed	wholesome

None of these are better or worse than the other, nor is this a comprehensive list. Choose two, three, or four of these—or countless other words that describe how you desire to feel—and let them fuel your movement forward. Just make sure they're your own. Which leads me to . . .

Mistake #3:
The goal isn't yours in the first place.

This mistake is more common than it ought to be. Chasing a goal based on someone else's desires means it never fully feels ours, and resentment builds quickly without our even being aware of it.

I was once in a relationship with a guy who loved body building. At the time, I would kill myself in the gym and restrict my food so much that nothing felt enjoyable. My adrenals were burned-out, and I didn't personally find any joy in my new muscles. But we talked about it so much I actually convinced myself that I would be crazy if I wasn't into it, too.

Even though I was "meeting my goals in the gym," life just kind of felt gray. What I didn't realize at the time (oh 20/20 hindsight!) is that the goal of looking like a lean fitness competitor wasn't genuinely my own.

When I stopped doing all of that—and again embraced things I love like Pilates, yoga, hikes, some weights, and an occasional slice of delightfully wholesome pizza—the world felt colorful again. I didn't stop being healthy, I just chose to do it in a different way. I decided that I'd take a rainbow world and slightly fuller thighs over maxing out my barbell squat any day of the week.

It wasn't the guy's fault—I had mistaken his goal as my own. And hey, I still love squats in my workouts, I just learned how to not badger myself over it. And to keep it real, I never have one slice of pizza. It's always two.

Mistake #4:
You forgot to paint the picture for everyday life.

Whoopsies. This gets us every time. Even if you avoid the three mistakes above, not painting your actionable goal into your everyday life can derail your results.

You may have heard of SMART goals in your work life, but just in case you need a recap: SMART stands for

$$Specific \quad Measurable \quad Achievable$$
$$Relevant \quad Time\text{-}bound$$

Setting SMART goals is a great start, but I hold that you also have to visualize how your daily actions reasonably fit into your current life situation. For instance, if you're a nurse who works 12-hour shifts, then "making a kale and fresh blueberry smoothie for breakfast every morning" might not be viable. If you don't have time to go to the store, or can't get up early enough, it's not going to happen.

In this case, a goal of "premake four days' worth of overnight oats to put in the work fridge for my 3 P.M. snack" would be more reasonable. We're going to get into this more in Parts II and III of this book, so stick with me.

THE ONE GOAL THAT SABOTAGES THE REST

Your goals are your own, so I don't want to place my own onto you. However, there is one goal that NO ONE should ever have, and that's the goal of perfection.

Perfection simply doesn't exist in the long-term, so including it in your goal plan is a surefire way to set yourself up for failure. As I mentioned before, consistency beats perfection every time. The dictionary definition of consistent is "acting or done in the same way over time, especially so as to be fair or accurate."

The definition of *perfection*—and I'm paraphrasing here—is a god-awful practice that women partake in, in which they meticulously torture, berate, and demean themselves and other people for the sake of an illusion that not only does not exist, but viciously teases your common sense and is at the epicenter of the worthiness crisis you experience every 15 seconds while maintaining a gleeful outer appearance. Or, more simply put: It's the opposite of nature's intention for you.

So, now that you know what not to do, let's talk about what to do. This is where it gets fun! I mean, not fun like those two slices of pizza I mentioned a few minutes ago, but I want you to keep reading so I'll make it as fun as humanly possible.

And by the way, if you're curious whether the information in this book applies to men, too, the answer is absolutely yes. Ninety-five percent of my blog traffic is female, so I generally speak to women when I teach. However, the glorious creatures known as men are always welcome here, too.

A STEP-BY-STEP PROCESS TO SET STRONG GOALS

1. List here, in your journal, whiteboard, phone, or anyplace that you wish the top three or more reasons you want to be healthy. The first things you write are generally high level and too abstract to turn into a goal, but they'll be a great starting place.

_____

_____

_____

2. Why do you want this? Think about a time in your life when you felt great. What words describe that feeling? Use the examples of desired feelings mentioned earlier (page 8) to get your juices flowing. Your *why* for wanting what you list in number 1 is your own. It can be something tangible, such as having enough energy to make it to 9 P.M., or intangible, such as feeling accomplished.

_____

_____

_____

3. How would achieving this desire or outcome make you feel? Keep going a few layers to find out that feeling you desire deep down. Take inventory of your desires and make sure they are your own. Don't rely on other people to define or achieve them.

_____

_____

_____

4. What outcome would support that feeling?

_____

_____

_____

5. What are the daily actionable steps that will support you in achieving that outcome? List as many as you can think of, and don't worry if you don't know these off the top of your head. This book will teach you what you need to do.

Daily Step 1
_____

_____

Daily Step 2
_____

_____

Daily Step 3 (and so on)
_____

_____

First comes desire, then the actionable daily goals. The outcome will be a natural by-product of the desire and daily actions.

It's okay to start with the outcome in mind if you're not sure what the desired feeling is, but work backward until you identify the desire. Remember, the desire is the fuel that will keep you engaged and committed to your daily actionable steps. Here are a few examples per the five questions above:

Example 1:

1. I want to have more energy in the morning while I'm with my kids.

2. Why? We all have more fun when I have more energy, and I want to enjoy my mornings more.

3. This would make me feel: more productive, more connected to my kids, more joyful in daily life.

4. An outcome that would support this would be to get to a point of going to bed before 9:30 P.M. so I can be asleep by 10 to get eight hours of uninterrupted sleep.

5. Daily actionable steps: low-glycemic dinner, no sugar or alcohol after 6 P.M., and creating a nighttime routine that quiets my mind and gets me ready to fall asleep more easily.

OLD GOAL: Have more energy.

New goals:

1. Six nights per week, eat a delicious low-glycemic dinner with protein and veggies.

2. Eat enough for dinner so I don't feel hungry and want to snack on sugar.

3. Write out my weekly dinner meal plan on Sunday and shop on Monday so I'm not caught off guard during the week.

4. Every night, take a melatonin and brush my teeth at 8:30 P.M. so I'm ready for bed at 9:30.

Example 2:

1. I want to lose weight.

2. Why? Because I will feel more confident in my clothes.

3. That would make me feel: confident, attractive, and possessing a huge sense of accomplishment for meeting my outcome. There was a point in my life when I weighed my goal weight and I felt energetic and confident. I would like that back.

4. An outcome that would support this would be to lose 15 pounds to help me fit into the clothes I want to wear.

5. Daily actionable steps: Putting an end to negative self-talk.

OLD GOAL: Lose 10 pounds.

New goals:

1. Meal prep five delicious low-glycemic breakfasts on Sunday so I can grab and go during the week.

2. Stick to my 10-hour eating window six days per week.

3. Log at least 10,000 steps per day.

4. Spend two minutes each morning writing down positive affirmations. (This is the most loaded line in this book. If weight loss is your goal, you can use these, but you'll come up with tailored daily actionable items as you learn here. Remember, these are just examples.)

Example 3:

1. I want my skin to break out less and heal more quickly when I do get a blemish.

2. Why? I could wear less makeup, itch less, and save money on all the skin products I buy.

3. This would make me feel: more confident when I meet with people at work and less worried about my skin. Relief from not feeling sometimes painful cystic acne.

4. An outcome that would support this would be to having a breakout-free month.

5. Daily actionable steps: Wash my face twice per day. Eliminate dairy to see if it helps. Drink enough water to hydrate and detox my skin.

OLD GOAL: Have better skin.

New goals:

1. Read labels carefully to eliminate all dairy from my food.

2. Diligently wash my face morning and night with an effective natural cleanser, followed by the right moisturizer and spot treatment when needed.

3. Drink at least 80 ounces of filtered water each day.

4. Track how my skin behaves in an app on my phone to see if there are any patterns with my cycle that I can prepare for each month.

Notice the differences in the desired feelings, outcomes, and daily actionable goals in the three examples above. It's also important to note here that you're free to reevaluate often. By nature, women are cyclical creatures.

We talked about the "F-word" (*freedom*) in the previous section, and it applies here, too. Just because you set a goal once doesn't mean that you're not free to reevaluate. Every now and again, reevaluate and reconnect with the purpose of your goals. Are they still yours? Are they still valid? Are they still helping you move toward your desired outcomes?

Now that you know how to set goals, there's one more simple, yet powerful, thing that you need to do, and that's to believe that it's possible.

Your beliefs shape your thinking, and your daily thoughts influence your daily actions. Your beliefs, or lack thereof, are the biggest barrier to achieving what you want. If you don't believe it's possible, it will never happen.

So take a moment to sit up, take a deep breath, and believe that you can create the habit of health. As Einstein said, "The world as we have created it is a process of our thinking. It cannot be changed without changing our thinking."

Having the belief that you can change your life for the better, even if other things have failed before, is the most critical first step to creating the desired outcomes you just identified. I believe in you. I know you have it in you to create positive change. Now I'm asking for you to believe in you.

This book will be your guide, and together with your belief that you can do it, you will change your life for good.

Chapter Summary

- Most people confuse goals with outcomes.

- If you don't understand the desire behind the outcomes you think you want, you usually do not reach your desired outcomes.

- Desires set the tone and fuel your actionable daily habits.

- Strong goals that support healthy habits come in the form of actionable daily steps.

- Outcomes are a by-product of connecting to desires and painting daily actionable steps into everyday life.

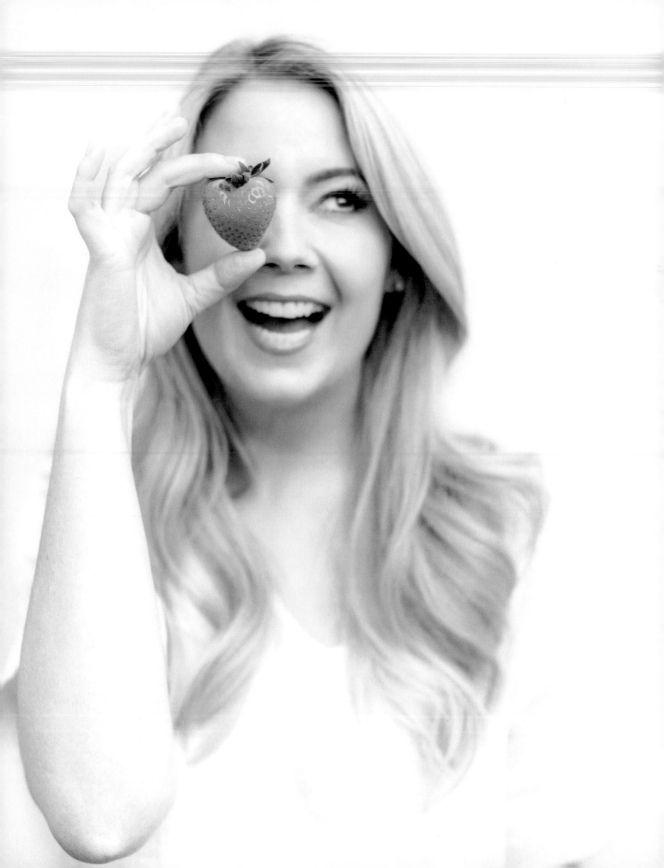

CHAPTER 2

The Qualitarian Way

Making the right choices, no matter how you eat.

t's time to get fired up. Like having to call the airline and wait on hold for an hour only to pay $390 to change a plane ticket you bought two days ago, followed by a call to your cell phone company about 15 extra charges for features you don't use, and rounding it out with a call to the cable company for tripling the price of your package, only to hear "that deal is only for new customers" fired up. (Because nothing brings out the best worst parts of you than airlines, cell phone companies, and cable providers.)

You've been lied to, and you should be mad. You don't need to *stay* mad—bless and release it, like forgiving the customer service agent who is just as frazzled as you are—but you do need to learn the real truth about real food. Specifically, how to get more of it, how to love the taste of it, and what minimally processed and packaged items are acceptable enough to allow into your food repertoire.

For the purposes of this book, when I talk about highly processed foods I mean foods that are so far from nature that they lack any nutrition. This includes items such as packaged, preservative-filled pastries and breads, meats with mystery ingredients, and lab-created foods.

Technically, any food changed from its original form would be considered processed, including my Cashew Basil Mint Pesto recipe (page 195), a smoothie made from wholesome ingredients, or a prepackaged item made with nutritious ingredients. These minimally processed foods are perfectly acceptable in the qualitarian way.

Unless you've been living under a rock for the past 10 years, you've probably heard that highly processed and packaged junk food is bad for you, and real food is good for you. Yet, I don't think most of us actually understand the lengths to which processed-food companies go to craft chemical combinations that make us addicted to their products. And don't think that this is just reserved for the big-bad-wolf companies out there. Some products that are labeled as "healthy" and found in health food stores do the same thing.

Scientists get paid big bucks to formulate flavors and combinations that set off a chemical response in your brain, one that keeps you coming back for more. Have you ever had a cheese puff and been satisfied with just one? Of course not. The flavor and texture of those things is carefully created to make you want more. On the flip side, have you ever wanted to eat more than one banana in a row? Not really. One usually does it (and that's what nature intended).

THE ONE LABEL
THAT FITS EVERYONE

Before we dive into the real truth about real food, I want to mention the one diet label that benefits everyone. We'll get into diet labels (vegan, paleo, or keto, anyone?) in the next chapter and whether or not it's a good idea to follow one, but in the context of real food, I want to introduce you to the concept of becoming a *qualitarian*.

A qualitarian is someone who may or may not follow a specific dietary plan, but who always evaluates the quality of food before consuming it. A qualitarian asks questions like, Where did this food come from? Are the ingredients naturally sourced? If it's animal-based, was the animal treated well? Is this high-quality food? Different people may have different answers to those questions.

The point is that—above all else—the quality of the food is the biggest factor in determining whether to consume it. The rest of this chapter will focus on becoming a qualitarian, regardless of what else you determine for

yourself, and helping you navigate all the food options available to you.

See, I told you this was going to be fun! And by fun I mean not restrictive or diet-y.

One of the biggest benefits of living the qualitarian way is that high-quality real food will generally lower chronic inflammation levels in your body.

Inflammation is your body's natural healing response. There are two types of inflammation: acute and chronic. Acute inflammation is something like swelling and scabbing that happens when you cut your finger.

Acute inflammation can also occur when you have a short-lived infection, injury, or toxins in your body. Your body goes into action to send blood and fluid to the spot the way moms flock to a Target sale, then heals the wound by closing it and forming a scab that eventually sloughs off.

Acute inflammation can also occur when you exercise and build muscle mass, which again is a good thing. Acute inflammation is generally helpful in terms of healing—it's what you want to happen when you hurt yourself.

Chronic inflammation, on the other hand, is not something you want hanging around in your body as it can have a negative impact on your overall health. Chronic inflammation occurs when cells and tissues just can't overcome the short-lived inflammation.

Chronic inflammation can be a result of consuming excessive amounts of sugar or eating poor-quality foods in general, as well as long-term exposure to harmful chemicals from things like beauty and cleaning products, air pollution, or toxic mold, just to name a few. It can damage your cells and organs, and lead

Qualitarian Commanding Principles

- Food grown from the earth is high quality. This can include both plant-based foods and animal-based foods. Even a carrot grown in low-quality soil contains more nutrients than a Dorito.

- The way in which food is grown can determine its quality. Plant-based foods and animal-based foods that are tainted during growth with harmful chemicals (such a glyphosate on crops), antibiotics, or hormones in animals, are not as high quality as those that are not, even though they come from the earth.

- Food that comes from poorly treated animals is not high quality. Animal welfare impacts the quality of food—both in spirit and in substance—whether a person is vegetarian or carnivore-friendly.

- Not all calories are created equally: 100 calories from packaged chocolate cake sets off a completely different hormonal response in your body than 100 calories from whole blueberries and nuts. As such, calorie counting does not create health.

- High amounts of added sugar of any kind degrade the quality of food.

- Some packaged and minimally processed foods can be high quality, but labels must always be read to understand what is in the package.

---

to chronic degenerative diseases including cancer, type 2 diabetes, and heart disease.

One reason chronic diseases are often called "lifestyle diseases" is because they can largely be prevented by living a healthy lifestyle. That's good news, and by following the steps in this book you can dramatically change your bad habits into healthy ones, and reduce the levels of chronic inflammation in your body.

Two eating styles that stand out in the qualitarian way are the Mediterranean diet and the Blue Zone diet, both of which are more eating styles than actual diets. The Mediterranean diet includes traditional foods found in eating habits of people in counties around the Mediterranean Sea such as Italy, Greece, and Spain.

So-called Blue Zones—coined by National Geographic Fellow Dan Buettner—are five areas of the world where people live the longest: Okinawa, Japan; the Ogliastra region of Sardinia, Italy; Nicoya Peninsula, Costa Rica; Ikaria, Greece; and Loma Linda, California. The longevity and high levels of lifetime happiness reported from the people in Blue Zones are largely attributed to their whole-food eating styles and daily movement.

Both the Mediterranean and Blue Zone ways include eating a plethora of vegetables, whole fruits, some (but not a lot) high-quality meat, reduced dairy, some type of fermented foods, and little to no added sugar. Neither of these eating styles requires strict labels. Rather, they focus on eating available foods that are close to nature.

SO, WHAT DOES REAL FOOD LOOK LIKE?

Here's the bad news: Over the past few decades, processed foods, and even processed "health foods," have taken over our grocery shelves and our kitchens.

But here's some good news: With a little inspiration and know-how, you can make real food the main focus of your daily eating plan. You can get back to basics with real food that is more convenient, less expensive, and even better tasting than processed foods.

Proteins

Quality dietary proteins come from meats (preferably naturally raised), eggs, and fish, as well as plant-based, protein-rich foods such as beans, lentils, and seeds. Some nuts, such as almonds, also contain a fair amount of protein. Some legumes, such as black beans and lentils, double as a protein and a good carbohydrate. Highly processed meats such as bacon and sausage are less desirable sources of protein because they often contain nitrates, preservatives, and fillers that you probably don't want to know about.

Good-quality protein powders such as grass-fed whey, pea protein, or hemp protein can also be part of a healthy eating plan.

Collagen protein powder has become quite the health food star as of late. Collagen is the most abundant protein in your body that weaves your connective tissues together. It gives your skin that youthful bounce and makes your hair and nails long and strong. It can also help heal the lining of your gut.

Nutrition-wise, collagen is not a complete protein (i.e., it does not contain all nine essential amino acids), so it should not be relied upon as your main source of protein. However, since it gives your body the building blocks to make more of its own collagen, it makes a fantastic addition to your smoothies, soups, or favorite hot drink for its beauty-boosting and gut-healing properties.

Proteins are chains of the amino acids that are the building blocks of your body. Protein satiates you, so if you often feel hungry or are hit with an urge to snack, try boosting your protein intake.

You need a moderate amount of protein to be healthy. I don't find it beneficial to ask you to count calories or weigh your food, but you should generally know how much protein you're getting, because women often don't get enough of it.

As a rough calculation, a good formula that will help you maintain a healthy body weight is 0.8 grams to 1 gram of protein per kilogram of your naturally healthy body weight. (Yes, we Americans need to use the metric system for a moment.)

That means if your naturally healthy body weight is 150 pounds (roughly 68 kilograms), 54 to 68 grams of protein per day will help you maintain a healthy weight. That's about 15 to

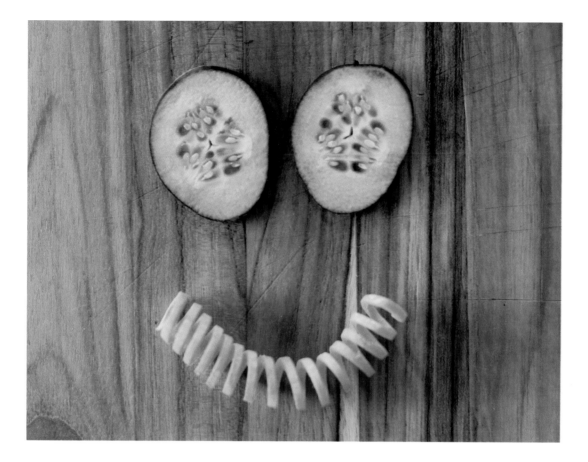

20 grams of protein in your main meals and some protein in your snacks, assuming you eat five times per day.

There's no reason for you to go onto a high-protein diet, because your body can convert excess protein into glucose, which raises your insulin levels and doesn't serve your health. This means you need to understand what "a moderate amount of protein" actually means.

Again, I don't want you to obsess about counting, but there are some things, like protein, water, and fiber, that you need to have ballpark goals for. Examples of ways to get about 20 grams of protein in one meal would

be one whole egg plus two more egg whites, scrambled; or one medium-size chicken breast; or unsweetened Icelandic or Greek yogurt with a few tablespoons of nuts or seeds; or one heaping cup of cooked black beans; or a high-quality protein powder blended in a smoothie.

Healthy Fats

Quality healthy fats can come from plant-based foods, including avocados; olives; extra-virgin olive oil; coconuts; tree nuts such as cashews, walnuts, and almonds; and seeds such as chia and flax.

Highly refined oils, such as vegetable oils, are undesirable sources of fats because they've been heated to the point of denaturing the oil and contain fewer nutrients than higher-quality options. The term *denatured* means that a food, in this case oil, is heated to a point that its chemical composition is changed, thus making it more difficult for the body to assimilate. Vegetable, canola, soybean, and other highly processed oils are often heated to the point of becoming denatured during the manufacturing process.

Real-food fats also come from animal sources, including milk, butter, ghee (clarified butter), eggs, and some cuts of meat. These don't work for everyone, as many people cannot tolerate the proteins found in milk and butter and avoid dairy, and some do not consume meat as a personal decision.

Whatever the source, healthy fats keep your cell membranes permeable, important to allowing nutrients in and waste out. They also help keep your skin hydrated and hair shiny—yes, fats are beautifying. Include healthy fats in all of your meals and snacks, and avoid "low-fat" processed foods, as they're usually stuffed with sugar to compensate for the lack of flavor.

Carbohydrates

Carbohydrates come from plants. Real-food, healthy carbohydrates include vegetables, whole fruits, whole grains (think whole rolled oats, rice, and quinoa), and legumes (beans and lentils).

Highly processed, and thus undesirable, carbohydrates come from grain flours. You know the culprits—bread, tortillas, pasta, pastries.

Nothing sabotages your healthy habits and

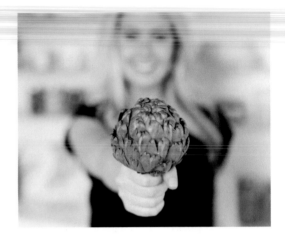

efforts more than nutrient-void, highly processed carbohydrates. Even breads or crackers labeled "whole wheat" or "whole grain" are usually still highly processed and raise your blood sugar levels to alarming rates.

Eating two slices of highly processed whole-wheat bread can elevate your blood sugar even more than two tablespoons of white table sugar! We'll talk more about blood sugar in the next chapter; just know that foods containing highly processed carbohydrates should be consumed in moderation or cut out altogether.

However, unprocessed carbohydrates, like the vegetables, whole fruits, legumes, and whole grains (if you tolerate them) mentioned above, are absolutely healthy and do not need to be cut from your eating plan. Just don't make highly processed carbs the main part of any meal, as they're mostly devoid of nutrients, contain excessive amounts of sodium, and can cause those blood sugar spikes. (And if you do eat bread, one made of a fermented sourdough starter, plus high-quality flour, salt, and water—just those four ingredients—is the healthiest choice.) Sprouted-grain breads made with wholesome ingredients can also be an occasional choice if you tolerate grains, but not the main event.

Instead, try one of the many wonderful wholesome alternatives to these items, such as brown rice pasta and Almond Flour Bread (page 190). You may be surprised how your taste buds will enjoy these, and your body will thank you.

Other highly processed foods—such as sugar-laden flavored yogurts, sugary drinks, canned foods loaded with sodium and preservatives, and condiments such as soy sauce—are full of sodium, excess sugar, and artificial preservatives. Simple swaps for these items will make a big difference in your health (see page 28 and the handy chart on pages 152–153 of the 28-Day Kick-Start Plan).

SUPERFOODS

You may have heard the word *superfood* before and wondered which foods actually qualify for this designation. It may seem like the food has to sound exotic (goji berries), be hard to pronounce (acai), or be the most expensive thing on the shelf (dragon fruit in the middle of the Rocky Mountains in December).

But the truth is that just about all foods from nature are "super." The humble black bean doubles as a protein and good carbohydrate, and is loaded with fiber, essential minerals, and B vitamins. Apples and bananas are superheroes loaded with natural hydration, antioxidants, and fiber. The same goes for just about anything in the produce section of your local store.

I also like to use the word *superfood* in recipes to remind my blog readers that a recipe is good for them. But don't be fooled into thinking that nature's abundant basics aren't just as good for you as a one-ounce $15 bag of the current "it" food in wellness.

Food is generally higher in nutrients when it's in season, so go for the freshest in-season food at the best price you can find.

SUGAR:
IT'S SNEAKIER THAN YOU THINK

By now you've heard that consuming excessive amounts of sugar is bad for you. But most people don't realize how sneaky companies have become at hiding sugar, especially in savory foods.

It's up to you to read labels carefully and watch out for hidden sugar. The World Health Organization (WHO) recommends consuming fewer than 25 grams of added sugar per day for women (35 grams for men),[1] and leading nutritionists and health experts agree.

However, I want to make one thing clear: Naturally occurring sugars in fruits and veggies do *not* count as part of that total, which means you can still enjoy sweet foods such as fruit smoothies without dipping into your daily allowance. WHO is referring to any sugar that is *added* to a food, including natural sweeteners.

If you eat any packaged or premade food, this 25-gram allowance adds up shockingly fast. You know your home renovation budget goes further when you DIY it a little, and the same rules apply here. If you make most of your own food, you can spread out your sugar budget with more than enough left over.

Most six-ounce flavored yogurts contain a whopping 20 to 26 grams of sugar, which is more than a Snickers bar, and more than your total daily allowance. Even savory foods can contain high amounts of added sugar; most store-bought marinara sauce contains 10 to 12 grams of sugar *per ½ cup serving*.

Sugar even hides in foods that seem healthy. Just as you can put lipstick on a pig, you can put vegan frosting on a cupcake but— you guessed it—it's still a cupcake. Manufacturers know that you're savvy and probably looking for sugar on the label, so they just simply rename it.

Here are dozens of other names for sugar that's still sugar . . . look for them when you read product labels:

Other Names for Sugar:

Agave nectar	Coconut sugar	Fruit juice concentrate	Organic cane sugar
Barbados sugar	Confectioner's sugar	Glucose	Palm sugar
Barley malt	Corn sweetener	Glucose solids	Powdered sugar
Barley malt syrup	Corn syrup	Golden sugar	Raw sugar
Beet sugar	Corn syrup solids	Golden syrup	Refiner's syrup
Brown sugar	Date sugar	Grape sugar	Rice syrup
Buttered syrup	Dehydrated cane juice	High-fructose corn syrup (HFCS)	Sorghum syrup
Cane juice	Demerara sugar	Honey	Sucrose
Cane juice crystals	Dextrin	Invert sugar	Sugar (granulated)
Cane sugar	Dextrose	Malt syrup	Sweet sorghum
Caramel	Evaporated cane juice	Maltodextrin	Syrup
Carob syrup	Fructose	Maltose	Turbinado sugar
Castor sugar	Fruit juice	Mannose	
Coconut palm sugar		Maple syrup	
		Molasses	

Remember, since the sugars present in real, whole fruits and veggies don't count toward the 25 grams of added sugar limit (35 for men) mentioned above, you can use whole fruits and veggies to add flavor, sweetness, and extra nutrition to your food. Just try to use the *whole* piece of fruit, not just the juice, as the fiber and extra water in the whole fruit are necessary to keep the natural sugars healthy.

If you like to hang out in the health and wellness space, you've probably heard people say that fructose (the sugar found in fruit) is bad for you. That's only a half-truth. When fructose is taken out of context (i.e., literally out of the whole fruit in the form of juice) and distilled down to just fructose, then it can be hard on your liver.

But keep in mind, fructose doesn't occur naturally on its own anywhere in nature. (High-fructose corn syrup and agave nectar are both processed, distilled forms of fructose and should be avoided.) The vitamins, minerals, fiber, and water in the whole fruit turn the entire package into one of healthiest options you can make.

A study of more than 6,000 women who were followed for six years showed reduced odds of depressive symptoms among those who ate two or more pieces of fruit per day, even after adjusting for factors including smoking, alcohol, body mass index, physical activity, marital status, education, energy, fish intake, and comorbidities.[2] (By the way, a comorbidity is the simultaneous presence of two chronic diseases or conditions in a patient. I had to look that one up, too.)

Have you ever tasted a ripe, in-season peach or some raspberries straight off the bush? No gummy candy or slushy can replicate that flavor. When at home, try unsweetened Greek or coconut yogurt with berries and a teaspoon of raw honey; it contains only 6 grams of added sugar (from the honey), so it's a much better choice than that whopping 26 grams in presweetened yogurt.

Or try a small apple with two tablespoons of unsweetened almond butter; no added sugar here! "Nice-Cream," a blend of frozen bananas that resembles ice cream, is another great, no-added-sugar dessert option. There are a lot of real-food options to satisfy your sweet tooth—check my website (elizabethrider.com) for even more ideas.

WHAT ABOUT SUGAR SUBSTITUTES?

Don't think you can just replace sugar with artificial sweeteners to tame your sweet tooth. It may be shocking, but marketers have once again not been fully truthful with you. Artificial sweeteners such as Splenda, NutraSweet, and Truvia aren't doing your health any favors. Studies have shown that people who use artificial sweeteners (e.g., by drinking diet soda or tearing into those colorful packets when they have their coffee) actually weigh more than people who don't use them.

Artificial sweeteners can create the same hormonal response in your body as sugar. Yep, you read that correctly. Adding two Splendas to your coffee can cause the same blood sugar spike as real sugar. Science is now understanding that just because something is zero calorie doesn't mean that your body doesn't perceive it the same way. It's best to just avoid artificial sweeteners altogether.

Now that I told you to stay away from added sugar and artificial sweeteners, you may be thinking, *Cool! I'll just use stevia instead.* Well, my friend, that's another misstep.

While natural zero-calorie sweeteners like stevia and monk fruit are fine to use occasionally, just like their artificial counterparts, they can still set off the same hormonal response as sugar. If you're trying to decrease your sugar intake, a few drops of one of these can help wean you off. However, don't rely on dropperfuls in your coffee every morning for the long haul.

The goal is to allow your brain to remember the joy of natural sweetness from real food, not trick it into believing something is sweet.

GRAB THE SEA SALT

I have good news: I'm going to tell you it's okay to eat salt. It's the sodium you have to be careful of.

You may now be thinking, *Wait, what?* So let's clear up some major confusion about the way we talk about salt. While the words *salt* and *sodium* are often used interchangeably, they are not the same thing.

When most people say "salt" in the context of food, they mean sodium chloride (NaCl), which is table salt. Sodium chloride (table salt) is 40 percent sodium and 60 percent chloride. But when we talk about healthy sodium levels, table salt is just one (small) source of dietary sodium. Other forms of sodium include saline, sodium benzoate, sodium bicarbonate (baking soda), monosodium glutamate (MSG), and a host of preservatives such as sodium nitrate.

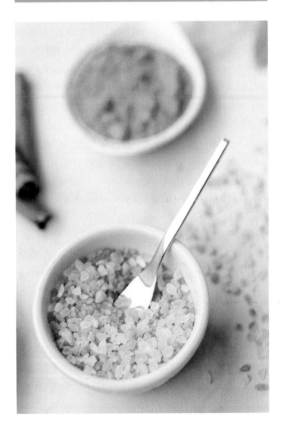

The majority of excessive amounts of sodium in the standard American diet—about 75 percent according to the U.S. Food and Drug Administration (FDA)—comes from eating packaged and restaurant foods, including food served at restaurants that you don't even know was packaged.

Only a small portion (11 percent) comes from salt added to food while cooking or eating at home.[3] I mention this because salt does wonders for flavoring your home-cooked food and can turn a bland meal into a gourmet dish.

So don't be afraid to cook with a little salt, as wonderful-tasting food will make you want to eat wholesome home-cooked meals more often. From a culinary perspective, salt enhances all flavors—even sweet ones, which is why you'll always see a pinch of sea salt in dessert recipes. The more you make your own meals, the more you can control the quality of your food and improve your health.

Most conventional table salt has the advantage of added iodine—called iodized salt—which came about in 1924 when the government realized that iodine deficiencies were causing high incidents of goiter (an enlarged thyroid).

However, in our modern times you can obtain the very small amount of iodine you need from fish, yogurt, eggs, sea veggies such as kelp, and vegetables that grow in iodine-rich soil. A good multivitamin will also contain some iodine, so it's no longer necessary to rely on table salt as your main source.

Since anticaking preservatives are often added to regular table salt, I prefer to cook with a high-quality unrefined sea salt to avoid these and other unnecessary additives. Sea salt is also sodium chloride (just like mainstream table salt), without the trace minerals stripped out.

The lesson here again is, when you do choose packaged food, read the labels and be alert for excessive sources of sodium other than salt. Remember, it's often the preservatives in packaged food (that don't even taste "salty") that contribute to excessive consumption of sodium.

Excessive sodium levels not only make you retain excess water weight, but they can raise your blood pressure out of the normal range, which can lead to stroke, heart disease, and heart failure.[4] Which leads me to one of the most important things you can do when developing your own Health Habit: Cook most of your own food.

THE ULTIMATE QUALITY CONTROL

When you cook and prepare most of your own food, you can control the quality of ingredients and amount of nutrition that you consume. This habit will of course depend on your lifestyle, but I encourage you to make your best effort.

It's helpful to remember that one of the reasons packaged food tastes so good is that the people who made it spent more time on the flavor than the nutrition! Try adding real flavor to your food to love it even more. Keep cinnamon, vanilla extract, chili powder, your favorite natural hot sauce, fresh herbs, sea salt, and other flavorful ingredients in your pantry and experiment with their use. They can make a world of difference when it comes to liking the meals you make.

Preparing your own food doesn't have to be hard. You can cook in batches, and find recipes that fit your time and budget.

One of the biggest advantages of cooking most of your own food is the amount of money you can save. When you buy prepared or packaged food, you're paying an extra convenience fee. Instead, batch-prepare at home and save.

If your budget allows, a food preparation and delivery program can be an equally great option if—and only if—the food is prepared in a homemade way and it's not simply repackaged convenience food. Be sure to vet the company and be sure that it's actually fresh and not a bunch of processed, preservative-laden food disguised as health food. That's no better than a TV dinner.

You'll pay extra for fresh-food services, but if that fits your budget, there's no shame in it. Ultimately, though, cooking and preparing your own food at home is both better on your budget and an act of self-care (we'll talk more about that in Chapter 6).

If you need ideas for cooking at home, check out the recipes at the end of the book and my website for loads of options to get you started.

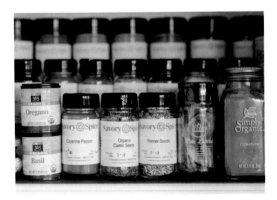

TAKING SOME HELP FROM MODERN CONVENIENCES

Now that I've alarmed you about added sugars, hidden sodium, and empty nutrition labels, let's come full circle and talk about how it's unreasonable to think that everyone can live in a world with absolutely no packaged food.

As I said in the introduction to this book, the best thing you can do for your well-being is focus on consistency, not perfection. We live in a fast-paced, imperfect world and there's nothing wrong with taking advantage of a few modern conveniences. Yes, you read that right. You're not failing at life if you rely on some packaged, minimally processed food—you just need to be smart about it. Here's how to do it.

First up, highly processed food should never be your first choice. You're proactive about your health (reading this book proves that), so this is not a surprise. What you might not realize is there's a wide definition of processed foods, from highly processed items like beef jerky containing only 10 percent beef, to hummus, which is technically processed but mostly just blended whole foods. Even homemade pesto is processed in your food processor.

In the context of this book, when I refer to processed food, I'm talking about highly processed food with low-quality ingredients. It's okay to pick and choose some healthier prepackaged items to make life easier, just look for minimally processed items with high-quality ingredients. These can be better than the alternative, which is not eating at all and becoming so hungry that you head to the nearest fast-food drive-through, or berating yourself for not being perfect.

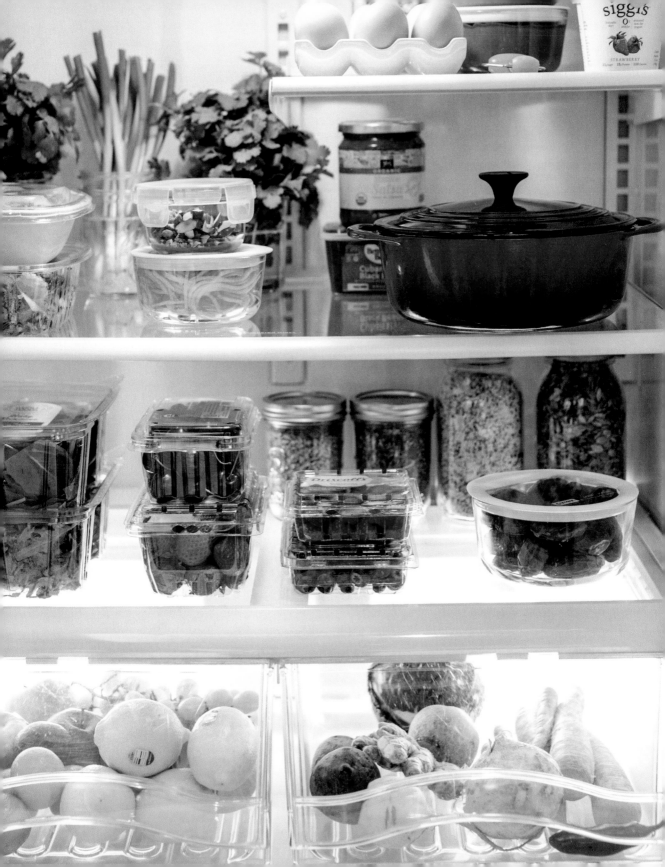

FOODS TO INCLUDE

Here are a few examples of foods that are technically processed but can still fit into your healthy eating plan:

Nut and seed butters, such as almond butter; they are even better if they have just one or a few ingredients.

Unsweetened or low-sugar Greek or Icelandic yogurt (if you tolerate dairy). Avoid any type of yogurt that is high in sugar or stabilizers/chemical thickeners, such as most dairy-free yogurts on the market.

Unsweetened nut milk or rice milk (look for carrageenan-free).

High-quality protein powders.

Condiments such as Dijon mustard or hot sauce made from high-quality ingredients. Just like everything, read the labels.

Real fermented veggies and krauts from the refrigerated section.

High-quality nitrate-free deli turkey or chicken, but be careful with these, as they are often excessively high in sodium and preservatives. Using them occasionally is totally fine and way better than a fast-food turkey sandwich.

Chicken stock or bone broth in a box; this can be your secret weapon when preparing a quick and delicious soup.

Foods that you've read the labels and feel okay about adding into your food repertoire.

FOODS TO AVOID

Then there is the list of ingredients to avoid. There is no scientific evidence that any of these support health. It's best to avoid them:

High-fructose corn syrup

Agave nectar

Trans fats (typically listed with the word *hydrogenated* in the ingredients list)

Artificial flavors

Monosodium glutamate (MSG)

Artificial colors (e.g., FD&C Yellow No. 6, Red No. 3)

Artificial sweeteners such as sucralose (Splenda), aspartame (Equal, NutraSweet), saccharin (Sweet'N Low), and others

Artificial preservatives like benzoates, sorbates, propionates, nitrates, nitrites, BHA, and BHT

Anything excessively high in sodium-rich ingredients

LET'S TALK BACKUP FOOD

Backup food is the stuff you keep around just in case you forgot to stock up on real food, or you're so tired that you just don't want to cook anything.

It's *not* meal-prep-Sunday food or make-ahead meals, it's the "sh!t-hit-the-fan-this-week" food you keep around to avoid "I'm-going-through-the-drive-through" emergencies.

We've all had days start with the best of intentions, then a work emergency hits or un-expected situation derails you: A contract falls through and you have 12 hours to write a new one to save everyone's year-end bonuses, or your kid falls off the monkey bars at school and you spend three hours in the ER waiting for stitches instead of making that homemade soup.

Backup food is your secret weapon against giving in and ordering pepperoni pizza from the delivery place that puts the same plasticiz-ers found in yoga mats into their dough (this happens!). Now, most people haven't put a lot of thought into this concept, so their backup food tends to be the candy in the bottom drawer, a bag of chips, take-out on speed dial, or the pint of ice cream in the freezer. But by getting into the habit of thinking ahead, you can get healthy.

When you don't have backup food on hand, you put yourself in the position of seem-ing to have absolutely no choice but to down a bag of Twizzlers. That is the hard way of doing things. When you have backup food on hand, you create an easier way to keep on track. Stay mindful of your habits and what you reach for by intelligent planning. By having healthy food options stashed away, you know you'll reach for them when you're stressed.

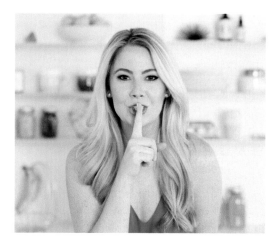

This means:

1. buying backup food that nourishes your body; and

2. being realistic about what you know you'll want.

For me, this means always having a high-quality pea protein powder in the pan-try, ready to be blended with half a frozen ba-nana and half a cup of frozen blueberries that I always keep in the freezer. Even if I've been traveling for 10 days, I can make this simple, healthy, and relatively inexpensive smoothie the morning after a long flight.

I also keep low-sugar chocolate peanut but-ter vegan bars in my computer bag, rice pasta in the pantry (it's come a long way in the last few years and now I prefer the texture over stan-dard versions), frozen fruits and veggies plus my favorite lentil soup in the freezer. I also stock organic frozen black bean burritos, because hey, you need backup food for period cravings, too.

Whatever it is for you, keep some good op-tions around for stressful times, as they will come.

Here are some backup food ideas if you need some inspiration:

- Frozen fruit, to be used frozen in smoothies or easily defrosted overnight in a glass bowl in the refrigerator

- Frozen veggies, such as whole edamame or a stir-fry mix

- Frozen homemade hearty soup (check out my website's recipe archive for loads of ideas)

- Frozen homemade avocado chocolate mousse, for when you want to eat dessert for dinner (see recipe on page 236)

- Frozen cashew cream, jarred no-sugar-added marinara, and brown rice noodles. Mix one part defrosted cashew cream to three parts jarred organic marinara for a creamy, decadent red sauce over brown rice penne noodles.

- Frozen organic burritos (I prefer the dairy-free ones)

- Frozen organic dinners, if you like them—but use caution with these; they usually contain high amounts of sodium or other undesirable ingredients. They're okay for backup food when needed, but not as your main go-to meals.

- Frozen homemade chili (check out the Game Day Chili recipe on page 234—it makes a fantastic family meal)

- A high-quality protein powder blended with frozen fruit can be a life-saver if you dig smoothies.

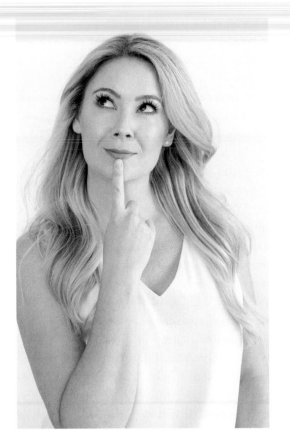

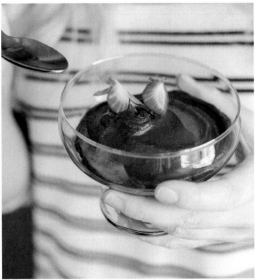

MULTIVITAMINS & SUPPLEMENTS: NECESSARY, OR EXPENSIVE PEE?

Multivitamins are a form of dietary supplements. A dietary supplement is a product that can contain vitamins, minerals, amino acids, herbs, or other substances that can be used to supplement the diet.

You may well ask, are dietary supplements such as multivitamins, fish oil, and vitamin D_3 real food? Nope! Even if a supplement comes from real food, the nutrients are still extracted—usually through hexane gas extraction—and it's still processed.

Supplements are well named, as they are meant to supplement your nutritional intake, not replace it. Since our physical body is made up of about 50 trillion cells, adding a little support is not only prudent, it's now even recommended by *JAMA: The Journal of the American Medical Association.*

High-quality supplements can fill in nutritional gaps to prevent deficiencies and help you optimize your body. And taking a high-quality multivitamin might be one of the simplest things you can do to improve your health.

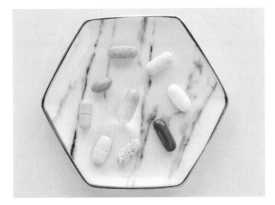

The initial Recommended Dietary Allowances (RDAs) for nutrients were first published in 1941 and were meant to prevent issues caused by acute nutritional deficiencies like scurvy. They've been updated since, but are still baseline requirements and don't provide optimal recommendations.

Just like with food, be a qualitarian with your supplements above all else. Whole food-based supplements that use hexane gas to extract the nutrients leave some of that hexane behind. This process is necessary . . . you can't just squeeze the beta carotene out of a carrot.

However, the FDA does not require companies to state sources, so it's best to do your research at the company and brand levels and buy only from companies you trust.

I recommend four dietary supplements to all of my clients:

1. high-quality multivitamin (remember, you get what you pay for)

2. an omega-3 fish oil supplement (unless you consume foods with omega-3s every day, which most people don't)

3. vitamin D_3 if needed (especially in winter months when you have little sun exposure)

4. a high-quality probiotic supplement (especially if you are not eating fermented foods regularly).

Supplements That Adapt to Your Needs

There are hundreds, if not thousands, of dietary supplements on the market. While we don't have space to cover every single one of them here, there is one category of supplements called adaptogens, or adaptogenic herbs, that I specifically want to mention.

Adaptogens do just what they sound like: They adapt to your needs. Used for thousands of years in Traditional Chinese Medicine and Ayurveda, they can help your adrenal glands make—or stop making—stress hormones as needed, thus helping your body adapt to its own individual needs. Examples include ashwaganda, ginseng, chaga, maca, and many others.

Adaptogens affect everyone differently. For instance, a naturopath once told me that ashwaganda gives him energy so he takes it in the morning. In my case, ashwaganda makes me so sleepy that when I first started taking it I thought something was majorly wrong with me. For more energy, I took it every day at noon for a week. I was literally falling asleep at 2 every afternoon. I called my doc and said, "It must be my thyroid," to which she replied, "We just checked that; start taking the ashwaganda at night and see what happens." Boom. Totally fixed and now I sleep better at night when I take it.

I also once tried maca, which is a South American root powder known for its healing and energy-giving qualities. This was way back in the day when I was just a few years into working in corporate America. I had hopped on the morning smoothie train and bought a tiny bag of precious maca powder for about $30 hoping it would give me a huge burst of energy to get through my morning.

The first morning, I added a teaspoon of maca to my smoothie and went on my way. The next morning, I woke up with big red bumps all over my legs. *Oh no, there must be a spider or bug in the bed*, I thought, which was completely plausible in my old house. I took apart all the bedding, washed everything, and went on with my day (surprise, I didn't find any spiders).

On day two, I added even more maca to my smoothie to help with the inflammation from these "bites." I thought I was brilliant. Day three rolled around, with even more welts all over my body, and as I'm making my smoothie it dawned on me: *Oh crap, I'm allergic to maca.*

I gave the bag away and my welts went with it. It was a good lesson to learn that just because something is natural, healing, or a superfood doesn't mean that it will jibe with your own biology.

Like everything you learn here to develop your own Health Habit, learn to use what works for you and leave the rest. Adaptogens are generally over-the-counter supplements, so do your research first and work with an Ayurvedic or Traditional Chinese Medicine practitioner, or another health-care provider, if you want to try one. As with all supplements, buy only from companies you trust and directly from the manufacturer or trusted source to avoid counterfeits.

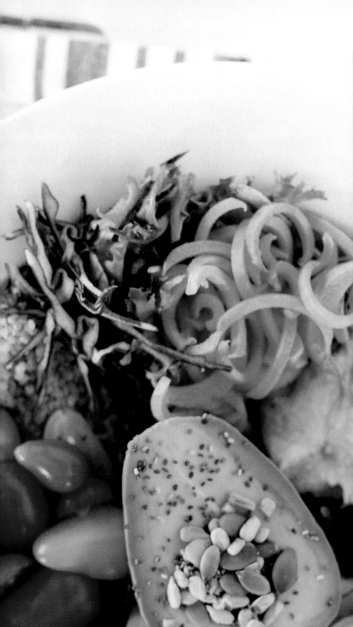

Chapter Summary

- Become a qualitarian and mostly consume high-quality foods.

- Read labels and avoid excessive or hidden sugar and artificial additives.

- Cook most of your own food by finding recipes that you enjoy.

- Choose packaged food wisely when you need modern conveniences.

- Have backup on hand.

- Take a high-quality multivitamin and other targeted supplements to fill in nutritional gaps as needed.

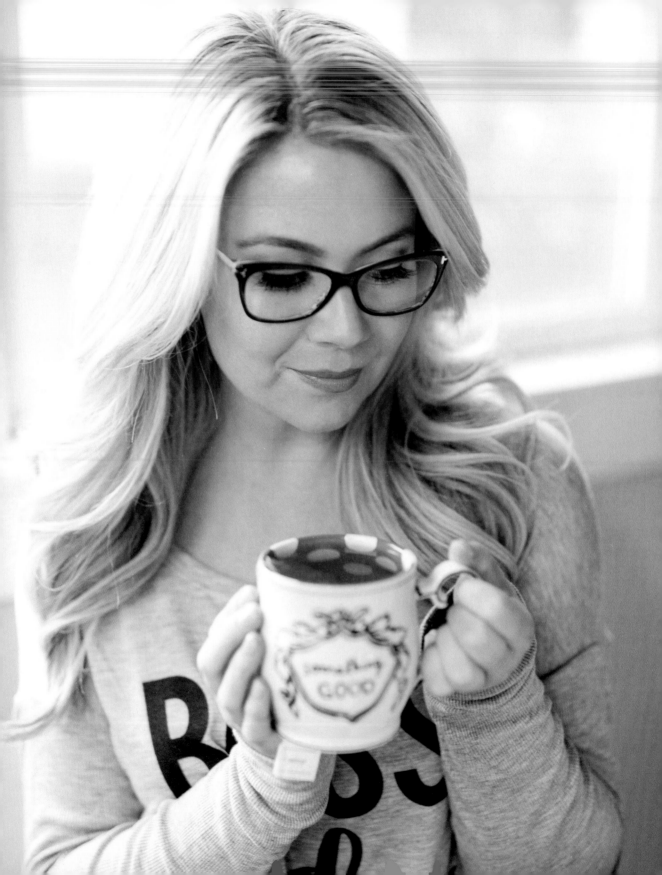

CHAPTER 3

Create an Eating Style That Works for You

You don't have to follow a specific diet,
but you do have to do this.

With the invention of the Internet, we have access to more information than any time in history. Want to learn how to host a cocktail party like Martha Stewart? Google it. Turn on your underground sprinkler system yourself instead of paying the landscape company $150 per hour to do it? Google it, and an exact step-by-step video pops up. Build a potato gun from scraps around your house? Easy-peasy! Just Google it.

With so much information available these days, you'd think that we'd be armed with the exact tools we need to know exactly how to eat. Yet, like some cruel twist of fate, we're more confused than ever about what to put in our mouths. Between the packaged food industry reaching more than $378 billion in the United States alone,[1] and the ability for anyone to say anything they want on the Internet, we have become entangled in quite a web of information—and misinformation.

In the last 10 or so years, the health industry has pushed consumers to choose a diet label. According to the latest Facebook feeds, chat forums, and celebrity endorsements, to achieve better health you have to be paleo, vegan, raw, keto, or gluten-free—or whatever diet-of-the-year happens to be on trend.

But here's the truth: Some fad diets work, for some people, but most do not. If you've ever had a friend who went paleo, vegan, or "just-eat-grapefruit" (or fill in the blank) and lost 10 pounds, then you tried it but gained 10 pounds, don't fret. It's not you. It's the diet. That specific diet doesn't work for your biology.

Moreover, you eat about 2,000 meals and snacks per year, give or take a few. I don't know a lot of people who can get something right 2,000 out of 2,000 times. One problem with diet labels is that if you mess up once you feel like you cheated, which puts you in a negative state of mind and exposes you to high levels of stress. Stress, not just food, can have a detrimental effect on your overall health.

You have to find the best way of eating for you, then make that into a habit. While the best way for you to do this may fit into one of these dietary theory camps, it might not.

Better yet, you can pull from many different ideas—vegi-Medditer-aleo—and create your own eating style that helps you look and feel your best. Not only that, your body is always changing, day to day, week to week, year to year. You might find you want more cooked food in the winter and cooling raw foods when it's hot out; lean vegetarian during some seasons and head toward meat in others.

In my opinion, aside from those shady types intentionally creating lies and counterfeit supplements for the sheer goal of profit, the biggest reason there's continual confusion about what to eat is that most people still don't understand that there isn't one right way for everyone. A blogger finds a way that works for her or him, raves about it online, and trumpets how "it's the *only* way." They're not intentionally misleading you, they're just sharing what they found works for them. The harm comes from when we buy into the idea that there's only one way to eat to be healthy, and when it doesn't work, we give up.

But that doesn't need to be the case.

TO LABEL OR NOT TO LABEL, THAT IS THE QUESTION

Before we talk about anything else, let's discuss whether or not you need to put a label on your eating habits. The first part of establishing a healthy eating habit that works for you in the long term is figuring out if you're an abstainer, a moderator, or a mix of the two.

The simplest way to do this is to consider both sides and determine which one gives you more freedom. As I talked about in Chapter 1, our lifestyle choices and healthy habits should ultimately make us feel free. If we don't, we will eventually resent them.

If you're a moderator, you're probably thinking, *But how can not doing something make you feel free!?* And if you're an abstainer, you're thinking, *Ah, yes, I feel more free when I don't have so many options. It feels better to be black and white about the habit.* You'll know which one you are based on how it makes you feel and whether or not you can best stick to your healthy habits.

Happiness and habit expert Gretchen Rubin writes:

You're a moderator if you . . .

—find that occasional indulgence heightens your pleasure—and strengthens your resolve

—get panicky at the thought of "never" getting or doing something

You're an abstainer if you . . .

—have trouble stopping something once you've started

—aren't tempted by things that you've decided are off-limits[2]

(Note: The exception to this is with an actual addiction to alcohol, drugs, or cigarettes. It's generally accepted that in these cases abstaining is the only solution.)

One of the biggest problems in the health and wellness world these days is that experts and coaches are trying to convert moderators into abstainers, or abstainers into moderators.

Not only does it not work, it feels terrible to be on the receiving end.

You have complete permission to know yourself, determine which approach resonates, and even be a mix of the two. Personally, I'm a moderator with a list of things I abstain from. Moderating qualitarian, perhaps? I eat well at home, and almost always choose a smoothie, salad, or protein and veggies dish when I'm out. Then occasionally I'll order a pizza with my family, and I can make a mean carbonara dish from scratch.

But no matter what, the *quality* of my food matters the most. I always abstain from highly processed breads or meats, fast food, or drinks with sugar in them.

Whether or not you decide to label your eating habits, the most important aspect of the food you choose is that it benefits you. We call this *functional food*, because it functions for you, not against you.

For example, pancakes made from nutritionally void bleached flour, white sugar, and denatured canola oil might taste good in the moment, but none of the ingredients have any nutritional benefits. Those pancakes don't function for you.

However, simple two-ingredient Egg and Banana Pancakes (see recipe on page 174) can be delicious flavored with cinnamon and vanilla and are loaded with protein, healthy carbs, vitamins, and minerals. This healthier choice delivers nutrition-boosting benefits and functions for your health.

Functional Food + The Qualitarian Way = More Health & Less Confusion.

When you combine the concept of functional food with becoming a qualitarian like we discussed in Chapter 2, you'll be headed toward more health and less confusion. Put another way: Functional Food + The Qualitarian Way = More Health & Less Confusion.

If you're an abstainer, diet labels can work for you. Words like *paleo* or *vegan* are music to your ears. If this is you, by all means label away.

For moderators, labels feel restrictive and absolutes like a life sentence. The 80/20 lifestyle (80 percent strict, 20 percent indulgence) really works for moderators, where abstainers are better off with an all-or-nothing approach.

Think about what approach is best for your pursuit of healthy eating habits and do that, no matter what labels others impose on you. Now let's move on to the most common topic that comes up in my conversations with clients: weight loss.

LET'S CHAT WEIGHT LOSS AND WEIGHT MAINTENANCE

I promised you that this isn't a diet book, and it's not. I debated even mentioning weight loss here and decided to add it because 1) I'm frequently asked about it, and 2) some of you just skipped ahead to this section because it's why you bought this book (You rebel, you! Promise me that you'll go back and read from the beginning because you need to understand the previous chapters to make this section effective).

For you rule followers who have read the book from the start, thanks for still reading. Now that we're all caught up, I need to share some thoughts about weight loss before we get into how to do it:

- You are not your weight.

- Your health is not all about weight. There are certain factors and biomarkers that weight can influence, but being healthy isn't all about being as skinny as possible.

- Your self-worth should not be tied to a number on a scale.

- Your wholeness and contribution to the world does not depend on how much you weigh.

- You don't owe anyone the goal of hitting a special number on the scale.

I deeply believe all of these things are true, and I hope you believe them, too. And, it's possible to believe those things and also know that you feel better at a certain weight and have a desire to achieve that weight.

Shaming women for wanting to lose weight is the same as shaming women for *not* wanting to lose weight. Your goals and desired outcomes are yours and yours alone, not your spouse's, significant other's, mom's, sister's, friend's, or trainer's. It's perfectly healthy to know that you feel more energetic and confident at a certain size or weight, and achieving that is worthy of establishing a Health Habit.

Think back to what we talked about in establishing goals (page 10). If weight loss is your desired outcome, shifting your internal dialogue and self-care are a huge piece of this. We'll cover those in this book soon, but for now I'll give you the basic facts you need to know about weight loss, because there's no such thing as one magic bullet that makes everyone lose weight.

5 TRUTHS ABOUT WEIGHT LOSS YOU NEED TO KNOW

Truth #1:

The quality of the calories you consume matters. Calories are a metric of energy, not nutrition, and all calories are not created equal. One hundred calories of potato chips sets off a completely different chain reaction of hormonal responses in your body than 100 calories of whole fruits and vegetables.

Empty calories from highly processed food generally burn faster than high-quality calories from nutrient-dense real food. In turn, these lower-quality calories can make you feel hungrier than before you even ate. In line with your new healthy habits as a qualitarian, the quality of the calories you consume should always be your first concern.

Truth #2:

If you consume more energy than your body uses, you will store that energy as fat. Highly processed carbohydrates and added sugars will fast-track you to overconsumption.

Truth #3:

If you burn more energy than you consume, your body will shed and release weight. This means creating a deficit in calories consumed to calories burned.

The biggest thing most people miss is that simply reducing calories is NOT always the best way to tip this balance. It's one way, but it's not necessarily the best way. It can backfire, as I explain below.

Truth #4:

Maintaining a healthy weight has far more to do with the food you consume than the amount of exercise you perform. Expecting to "exercise away" excess consumption of energy (food) will lead to a lot of frustration.

Truth #5:

If you're within 5 to 10 pounds of your goal weight, then weight loss might not be what you're after. You may simply need to change your body composition (e.g., build more muscle while losing a little fat); if you change your body composition, you may drop one to two sizes but you'll weigh the same on the scale.

Per these five truths, consuming fewer calories than what your body burns will lead to weight loss. However, that's not as straightforward as it sounds.

The oversimplification of "eat less, exercise more" leads to confusion and a whole lot of frustration because there are a variety of factors other than calories that influence how your body uses energy.

Your hormones—specifically insulin, ghrelin, leptin, cortisol, and thyroid hormones—your lean muscle mass, the quality of food you eat, the amount you move in a day, your stress levels, and some genetic factors all affect how much you will burn. Simply counting or restricting calories can backfire, because reducing calories consumed, or consuming poor-quality calories, can also change the rate at which your body burns those calories.

And don't blame your genes; your lifestyle has much more to do with your weight than your heritage. The field of epigenetics has shown that lifestyle choices can turn genes "on and off" (i.e., change the way they are expressed).

If you notice familial trends—like everyone in your family is overweight—it's possibly because you grew up with the same examples of lifestyle habits and developed the same emotional patterns, not just because of your genes. I mention this to remind you again that you are the master of your own fate. You have control over your lifestyle to set healthy habits that can ultimately express those genes in a different way (phew!).

An unhealthy calorie deficit comes from starving yourself, overexercising, extreme dieting, or eating lab-created "low-calorie" packaged food. This is generally not sustainable. The sensations of hunger, toxic burden, and obsession will make you feel miserable, and can potentially even slow down the rate at which your body uses energy, working against your desire to burn more calories than you consume.

Moreover, food is information because your cells talk to each other. This phenomenon is

But What about the Scale?

You might be wondering if you should weigh yourself. Here is my take: From a clinical perspective, most practitioners agree that weighing yourself once per week (right when you wake up, at the same time of day and under the same conditions to control variables) provides important information for you to understand where you're at and keep you on track. You do not need to weigh yourself every day. Once a week gives you a more accurate measurement as your hormones, monthly cycle, stress, and meal choices can cause slight fluctuations. However, if the scale triggers any type of dysmorphia or disordered behavior (for example, not eating), or if you have a history of an eating disorder, then it's best to say goodbye to the scale.

Nutrients and combinations of nutrients in food signal your cells to take certain actions (aka cell signaling). This means that the information in whole rolled oats and blueberries with a small amount of raw, enzyme-rich honey gives your cells different (better) information than the nutrient-void flour and processed sugar in a prepackaged blueberry muffin.

A healthy deficit can be created by filling up on nutrient-dense, quality food (it typically burns more slowly!) to keep hormonal responses on track, crowding out empty calories from highly processed carbs and sugar (I'm looking at you, breakfast pastries and packaged breadsticks), reducing stress (even the good kind), and getting your 10,000 steps in each day (we'll talk more about these in Chapter 6: no gym membership required).

A healthy deficit will leave you feeling satisfied, energetic, and—dare I say it—healthy without feeling like your new healthy habits are too hard.

known as cell signaling. Every time you eat—or more accurately, every time you digest a certain food—the combination of nutrients you absorb allows your cells to talk to each other.

As Dr. Mark Hyman says, "Some calories are addictive, others healing, some fattening, some metabolism-boosting. That's because food doesn't just contain calories, it contains information. Every bite of food you eat broadcasts a set of coded instructions to your body—instructions that can create either health or disease."

LOW-FAT OR LOW-CARB FOR WEIGHT LOSS?

A recent study out of Stanford University School of Medicine has finally solved the low-carb or low-fat debate for good.[3] It's a draw.

Yep, that's right. They both work equally well. The study recruited 609 participants between the ages of 18 and 50. About half were women and half were men. All were randomly placed into one of two dietary groups—low-carbohydrate or low-fat—and each group was instructed to maintain their diet for 12

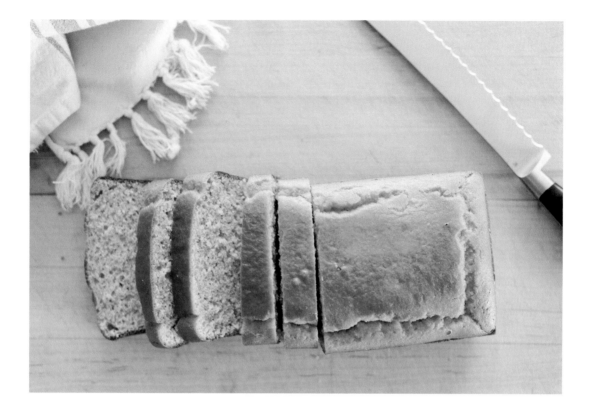

months. By the end of the study, everyone had lost an average of 13 pounds, with no significant differences between the two groups.

In my view, the most important part of this study is that each group was instructed to eat real (or very minimally processed) food. Based on claims from hundreds of fad diets, how could this be? Each group has die-hard fans praising the merits of their program while demonizing the other.

The reason it's a draw is simple: Both styles of eating reduce sugar, limit highly processed carbohydrates (and highly processed food in general), and encourage eating a plethora of fruits and vegetables. Both groups also consumed a moderate amount of protein while on

the study. The same study also noted, "On both sides, we heard from people who had lost the most weight that we had helped them change their relationship to food, and that now they were more thoughtful about how they ate."

A note of caution: The people in the low-fat group still ate some healthy fats, and their carbohydrates came from whole food sources, including vegetables, whole fruits, and legumes (beans, peas, and lentils), *not* croissants and double-mocha frappuccinos.

Trust me, I secretly wish I could live on a high-carb, bagel-for-breakfast-lunch-and-dinner diet and stay healthy, too, but that's not the case. In my opinion, this study highlights that one reason why people lose weight and gain health when they go hard-core paleo, vegan, or other diet du jour is because they are focusing more on real food that is nutrient-dense and slow burning, not necessarily because of the diet guidelines themselves. These strict diet labels can certainly have benefits and allow the gut to heal over time; however, it may be the focus on real food, not the label itself.

AN ALTERNATIVE TO WEIGHT LOSS

I want to explore again the concept that if you're within 10 pounds of your ideal weight and have a healthy body mass index (BMI), then a change in body composition (i.e., how much lean muscle mass versus fat you have on your body) may be what you're really after.

You can check with your health professional or go online to find a simple BMI calculator, as long as you know your current height and weight. Keep in mind that BMI is not a perfect measure of health because it doesn't take into account that muscle weighs more than fat by volume.

If you already engage in muscle-building activity, your BMI may read in the overweight range when really you just have more muscle than the average person. However, if you currently exercise a moderate amount doing mostly walking or cardio activities (or not at all), then the BMI chart will give you a decent picture of whether or not you're at a healthy weight for your height.

If you're within the normal range of your BMI for your height but want to be smaller or don't love your shape, increasing muscle mass will help you shrink and appear to lose weight. Muscle weighs more but takes up less space than fat, so it's possible to put on muscle and be smaller but weigh more. This is another reason why it's so important not to obsess about a number on a scale.

If you have 20 or more pounds to lose, then general weight loss, which is still mostly fat loss, may be what you're after. But if you're close to your ideal weight and want to feel tighter, add resistance training and weights to your exercise routine. Since I'm not a personal trainer (and my editor keeps telling me to stay on track), I can't guide you on this, but from my own experience, hiring a trainer to teach me how to lift weights was one of the best things I've ever done to maintain my happy weight.

You don't have to be a gym rat; I've never had the need to be in a fitness competition (but if that's your goal that's super cool—I admire your dedication). For most of us, just two or three 45-minute sessions a week of weights can help build muscle, burn more fat, and reduce a few inches, even as the number on the scale stays the same. You get more bang for your buck with your time in the gym, so get off of cardio machines and into free weights and resistance training.

For example, I'm five feet eight inches tall. When I have periods of time without strength training—generally because I'm traveling a lot or just want a break—I usually even out at about 145 pounds, which is a size 6 on my frame, even with clocking 10k steps per day from walking, yoga, or doing cardio.

On the flip side, which is where I like to live, when I'm consistent with strength and

Weight-Loss Quick Tips

We cover each of these topics in this book:

- Eat low-sugar meals and snacks, regardless of what type of eating style you follow (see page 44).

- Consider using time-restricted eating—a type of intermittent fasting—in your daily meal plan (see page 46).

- Consume no more than 25 grams of added sugar per day. Regard this as your budget and use it wisely; 25 grams is your max budget, so try to consume even less as you develop your Health Habit (see page 63).

- Aim for consuming roughly 15–20 grams of protein in your main meals three times per day. That's still considered a moderate amount of protein and will help you feel more full, and build or maintain lean muscle mass (see page 18).

- Get your gut microbiome in check by eating fermented foods, taking a probiotic, and consuming whole foods (see page 49).

- Burn more calories than you take in, not by restricting calories but by eating low-sugar quality food, taking 10,000 steps per day, and getting quality sleep (see page 38).

- Have your thyroid and vitamin D levels checked at your next doctor's appointment. Work with your health-care provider to get them into optimal ranges (see page 71).

- Consider adding more lean muscle mass to change your body composition with strength and resistance training (see page 42).

- Bookend your day with self-care to center yourself, so you'll want to do all of the above things without going crazy. Learn more about this method in Chapter 6.

- Remember that you are not your weight, and you don't owe anyone a number on a scale. Set your desired outcomes based on how you want to feel, not by outside pressure or standards. No one looks like a photoshopped supermodel in real life, so just let that pressure go.

resistance training, I usually weigh 146 to 150 pounds but am a size 4. I weigh more on a scale at a size 4 than I do at a size 6, because muscle is heavier than fat but takes up less space. I also eat more at my strength training size 4 because muscle needs more fuel.

More food, smaller pants, and strong legs make the three times a week I lift weights a joy and a worthwhile part of my Health Habit. These don't have to be your desired outcomes or goals, but if they are, I wanted to share those numbers with you for reference so you're not mistaking weight loss with body composition changes.

BASICS THAT
BENEFIT EVERYONE

You don't have to label your eating habits, but you do need to understand the fundamentals of how food affects your body. Whether you want to lose weight, or just simply feel better, be more energetic, and take better care of your health, the solution isn't another crazy-restrictive fad diet.

It's getting back to basics that work, and building these basics into your everyday habits. Along with becoming a qualitarian and understanding whether or not you're an abstainer or a moderator, these basics will help you stay on track to developing healthy habits that can fit into any eating style you choose to follow.

The Glycemic Index:
What You May Not Know

You've probably heard of the glycemic index before, but you probably don't know the whole story. You see, although the glycemic index has been taught for decades, most instructors didn't realize that what's low glycemic in one person might not be low glycemic in another. And vice versa. Yep, that's right. The same food can affect your blood sugar differently than it affects another person's. But why is this so important?

This distinction is critical to your health because most people who develop type 2 diabetes or other blood sugar disorders live with the condition for years—or decades—before it's diagnosed. You might think you're too young or that diabetes wouldn't happen to you

. . . and you'd be wrong. Even if you're at a healthy weight, you're at risk. But before we move to blood sugar issues, let's back up just in case you need a refresher.

The glycemic index rates foods based on how quickly they can cause your blood sugar to rise.[4] Foods low on the glycemic index cause a nice slow rise in your blood sugar, which makes you feel good and have optimal levels of energy.

High-glycemic foods, on the other hand, provoke rapid spikes and dips in blood sugar levels, which can make you feel hungry, moody, and low in energy.

A separate measure, called the glycemic load, also measures how quickly the food makes glucose enter the bloodstream and how much glucose it can deliver. This gives you a slightly more accurate picture of a particular food's impact on your blood sugar.

For instance, watermelon is technically high on the glycemic index, but because it contains so much water and very little carbohydrates it has a very low glycemic load. High-glycemic foods include the obvious offenders such as cookies, candy, and brownies. Items made from processed grain flours, like regular white flour or wheat flour, are also typically high glycemic.

Low-glycemic foods include most vegetables, most whole fruits, legumes (beans, peas, and lentils), nuts, meats, fish, eggs, and some whole grains. Consuming only foods that are low on the glycemic index will help stabilize your blood sugar levels, even out your moods, and release excess weight from your body.

While the glycemic index is an effective tool to create better health, here's the kicker:

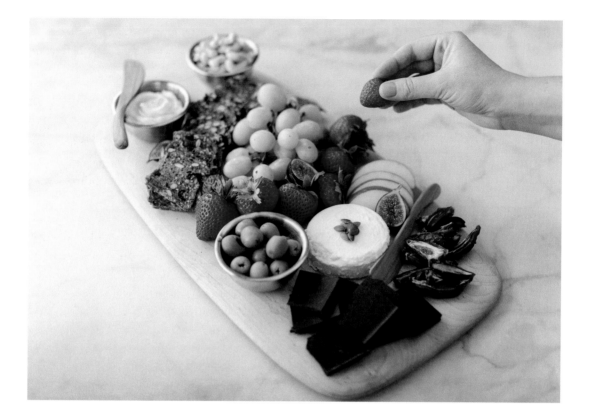

It's just a reference chart used for predictions. It doesn't tell you how high *your own* blood sugar will go after eating a certain food. And since everyone's biology can react differently, you need to use a blood glucose monitor to understand how your own biology responds.

For example, I know when I order pad thai (my favorite takeout, made with rice noodles, green onions, eggs, tamarind, and veggies), 30 minutes after I finish my meal my blood sugar spikes up to 160. Even though this meal is gluten-free, dairy-free, and appears relatively healthy, there isn't enough protein in the dish to slow down the absorption of the carbohydrates from the rice noodles and veggies.

If I order that same dish with chicken, my blood sugar hovers at about 128 (within the normal range). But remember, this is my experience. A friend did this same experiment with me on the same night, and while my blood sugar went to 128, hers spiked all the way to 180, even with the chicken.

The only way you can know how this meal affects you is to test it yourself. I don't eat pad thai that often, but now I know how I can enjoy it from that restaurant without having to worry about my blood sugar levels. However, since no two restaurants use the same recipe, you'll have to experiment when you eat at different places.

You can buy a blood glucose monitor at just about any pharmacy for around $30.

The test strips are what cost more, but you can start with the smallest pack available (usually around $20). We'll talk more about blood glucose (blood sugar) levels in the next chapter, but for reference here, most functional medicine practitioners look for a fasting blood glucose (upon waking) of 90 or less (but not below 70, which is too low). Thirty minutes after eating, it should remain under 135.

If you find yourself outside of the normal range, focus on constructing low-glycemic meals and snacks. To do this, simply combine a protein and/or fat with a good carbohydrate.

If you find fruits and vegetables quickly spike your blood sugar out of the normal range, eat the protein and/or fat *before* the carb, not at the same time. For example, a nutritionist friend of mine told me that she loves to visit her family's orchard back East to pick fresh cherries. She's been in the habit of testing her blood sugar, and she suspected a big handful of cherries on their own would cause a spike. She was right; 30 minutes after eating the cherries her blood sugar was over 175! The next day, she repeated the experiment but ate two slices of nitrate-free organic turkey before she ate the cherries. Sure enough, 30 minutes later, her blood sugar remained under 135.

What's important here is that she didn't demonize the nutrient-filled fruit, forgo the delightful pleasure of tasting fresh cherries, or miss out on family time, all of which contribute positively to her health. She stayed on top of her numbers and simply combined

———

Time-restricted eating does not mean starving yourself.

———

the cherries with some protein to remedy the situation.

I found her story interesting so I bought some cherries myself. I ate them without any other food on an empty stomach and 30 minutes later my blood sugar was 132, still well within the normal range. I suspected that would be the case because I know that I feel great when I eat fruits and veggies and sluggish if I eat an excessive amount of fats, even healthy ones.

My body tends to do better on real, natural carbohydrates as opposed to a paleo style of eating. This just goes to show that we all respond to foods differently, so it's important to get that blood glucose monitor and see for yourself. Try and test every morning and after lunch and dinner for a week; if you're in the normal ranges, then no need to keep on testing. Just repeat that experiment every six months to a year to make sure you're on track.

I'm going to teach you how to get intimate with your blood glucose levels in the next chapter, but first, let's cover a few more ways to easily develop daily healthy habits that will serve you for life.

A Fast Way to Improve Your Health

Intermittent fasting has been used for centuries to improve health. It's simple, effective, and easy to follow . . . when done right. Intermittent fasting isn't about eating less, it's about eating smarter. It works by allowing your body to lower insulin levels for longer periods of time. This helps prevent insulin resistance and keeps your body in a fat-burning zone longer.

With what I consider the least sexy, most unappealing name ever, the label "time-restricted eating" is here for the win, and although the name alone makes food-loving women want to hide under their desks, it's something you need to know about. I'm going to stick with the name now because that's what the scientists call it, but later on I'll refer to this as "your eating window" because that sounds much more tolerable. And trust me, this is way easier than it sounds at first glance.

Time-restricted eating is a form of intermittent fasting where meals are consumed within a specific period of time. A popular and extremely effective form of this way of eating is an 8-hour eating window, then fasting for the remaining 16 hours of the day, called 16:8. Generally, this is done every day or almost every day.

Benefits of time-restricted eating can include:

* Improved mental clarity and concentration
* Increased energy
* Weight and body fat loss
* Improved lean muscle mass
* Balanced blood glucose (sugar) levels
* Improved fat burning

Along with everything else I teach in this book—you guessed it—you get to find an eating window that works for you. Here are a few examples:

SAMPLE TIMEFRAME	EATING WINDOW
8-hour eating window, with 16 hours of fasting between dinner and breakfast the next day	8 A.M. TO 4 P.M., 9 A.M. TO 5 P.M., OR NOON TO 8 P.M.
10-hour eating window, with 14 hours of fasting between dinner and breakfast the next day	8 A.M. TO 6 P.M. OR 10 A.M. TO 8 P.M.
12-hour eating window, with 12 hours of fasting between dinner and breakfast the next day	7 A.M. TO 7 P.M.

The most important thing about utilizing time-restricted eating is giving your digestion and insulin levels a rest between dinner and breakfast the next day. A slow trickle of food or drinks (except water) up until you go to bed will keep your insulin levels high, which can deplete your energy, affect your sleep, increase inflammation in the body, and make it difficult to lose or maintain weight.

I find most women do well with a 9- or even 10-hour eating window for optimal health. Most days I personally have breakfast around 9 A.M. and dinner between 5 and 6 P.M., which has garnered me the loving nickname "blue-plate special" from some of my girlfriends. But the joke's on them because

Do I Need to Detox?

Detoxing is built into the magnificence of this miracle we call a human body. Your lungs, skin, liver, kidneys, circulatory system, digestive system, and lymphatic systems work tirelessly, 24/7, on autopilot (thanks, autonomic nervous system!), efficiently ridding your body of toxins and metabolic waste. They are pretty darn good at it.

Going on a detox or doing a cleanse doesn't automatically make your detox organs any better than they already are. However, lessening the burden on them by decreasing the toxic inputs can allow your body to use some of that saved energy to do more healing. But just doing it for three to five days isn't necessarily a big win. Lessening the burden over time, as part of your Health Habit for the long haul, by following the lifestyle outlined in this book will help the most.

One significant benefit to doing a short-term cleanse or a detox is that it can reset your habits and your expectations of how you follow your habits. This can be tremendously beneficial to set you on a good path, and is something I do a few times per year.

If it's helpful for you to do a cleanse or detox to kick-start better habits, then by all means do it. That's why I give you a 28-Day Kick-Start Plan at the end of this book. But please don't starve yourself for prolonged periods of time, as that doesn't benefit you in the long term.

restaurants usually have better prices from 4 to 6 P.M., and I sleep much more soundly when I stick to this practice.

If you're new to this concept and generally snack before bedtime, even shortening your eating window to 10 or 11 hours will have health benefits.

Remember, time-restricted eating does not mean starving yourself. I can't emphasize that enough. The biggest mistake people make when trying intermittent fasting is not eating enough.

It's not about eating less, it's about eating the same amount but in a shorter time period. So be sure to eat enough at dinner so you don't feel hungry before bed. Sticking to this type of intermittent fasting is safe to do every day, and has proven benefits if it's followed at least five days per week, which goes back to your goal of consistency, not perfection, in establishing your Health Habit.

When you have an occasional night on the town, just have fun! Don't miss out on the benefits of a loud-and-late dinner with friends. (Or, if you're a social introvert like me, going out with friends then coming home early because you love them but want to be alone and enjoy a 9 P.M. black bean burrito while you catch up on Netflix.)

And, for the love of God, just enjoy Thanksgiving Day without freaking out about the feast. Aim for high-quality foods and ingredients on special occasions, but bless and release it all on a big day. One meal outside of your eating window every once in a while isn't going to sabotage you, it's what you do after (i.e., getting back on track the next day, and the next, and the next) that matters.

Moderators, you will be delighted with those statements. Abstainers, I know you just had a mini panic attack. It's okay, breathe. You don't have to stick to time-restricted eating only five days per week. It's healthy to do every day and never miss a beat, if that feels better to you. Pregnant women or individuals with a history of disordered eating should abstain from all types of fasting. People with diabetes or cancer should consult a health-care provider before engaging in any type of fasting.

Get Your Gut Right

Your digestive tract is one big ecosystem, made up of hundreds of diverse bacterial species. This ecosystem, including the microbes and their DNA, is called your gut microbiome. In fact, you have more bacterial cells in your digestive system than cells in your body—about three to five pounds worth.

The gut microbiome is a subset of your body's microbiome. Both inside and out, your body hosts a huge array of microorganisms on your skin, in your organs, and circulating through your entire system. A lack of good bacteria in your digestive system can lead to a variety of digestive disorders, including leaky gut, small intestinal bacterial overgrowth (SIBO), or another type of gut dysbiosis such as an overgrowth of candida. For the purposes of this book I'm going to give you some overly simplified explanations of these, since we're not sitting in a medical conference and I'm trying desperately hard not to sound boring.

Leaky gut is a condition in which unhealthy processed foods, preservatives, high amounts of sugar, pharmaceuticals, lack of good bacteria, and even stress can cause the lining of the small intestine to develop microscopic holes. Particles of food or other things can then pass through these tiny openings and into your bloodstream, where they are not supposed to be.

As an example, think of it like stretching plastic wrap over a bowl of water. If you turn the bowl of water upside down, no water should come out. But if you poke a few pinholes in the plastic, water will drip through. The plastic wrap in this case is like the lining of your small intestine. It shouldn't have any holes.

Your small intestine isn't smooth like plastic wrap, rather it's covered by tiny thread-like projections called villi that increase your intestinal absorptive surface to somewhere in the neighborhood of 160 square feet! That's a lot of area to absorb the nutrients (and toxins) from your food. In addition to the culprits I listed above, refined grains, gluten, sugar, dairy, genetically modified organisms (GMOs), pesticides, and artificial sweeteners can all contribute to leaky gut.

Your gut microbiome—a sub system of your overall microbiome—is the collection of good and bad bacteria in your digestive system. It's responsible for keeping your health in balance. SIBO is a condition where normal bacteria are misplaced in your digestive tract, throwing everything out of balance. This can come from bacteria that is supposed to live in your colon working its way backward in the digestive tract (yikes!) and making itself at home like your unemployed brother-in-law. It's unwelcome in the small intestine and needs to get kicked out to do its real job back in the colon.

But the goal isn't to get rid of all bacteria—that's impossible and we need it—but rather to get the bacteria back into balance. This can be accomplished by introducing good bacteria via fermented foods and probiotics, and eliminating the root cause of the dysbiosis, including processed foods, foods that you may have a sensitivity to, excess sugar, excessive use of pharmaceuticals, and stress.

Gut dysbiosis is an imbalance of bacteria somewhere in your digestive tract, for example your stomach, small intestine, or colon (large intestine). It's broadly defined as any change to the composition of resident commensal communities relative to the community found in healthy individuals.[5] In layman's terms, it means your gut bacteria is out of whack.

Candida is one type of bacteria that lives in your gut. It loves sugar and feeds on it like a sleep-deprived mom feeds on coffee. When too much sugar is present in the gut, candida goes hog wild feeding on it, growing and taking over. You may have heard people say, "I have candida," which is correct for us all. A little candida is normal and supposed to be there, a lot can cause an imbalance (dysbiosis) and is a problem.

In many cases leaky gut, SIBO, or most types of gut dysbiosis can be healed by removing all processed sugar and preservatives from your regimen in combination with an elimination diet and/or implementing a gut-healing protocol. These digestive disorders can cause painful bloating (feeling like you look pregnant when you're not), uncomfortable or uncontrollable gas, loose stool, autoimmune conditions, or even food allergies or sensitivities.

An elimination diet does not have to be a death sentence for a certain food group. The real goal of an elimination diet is to pinpoint if a food is causing problems for your health, then heal the condition to be able to reincorporate the food.

> ## An elimination diet does not have to be a death sentence for a certain food group.

If you have an actual allergy then yes, you will probably have to eliminate the food forever. But if you eliminate a food to heal a food sensitivity or a gut condition, you can usually reincorporate high-quality versions of that food back into your meals, which was the case for me with dairy. I suspected leaky gut, so I decided to diligently remove dairy from my diet about five years ago, and my skin magically cleared up—especially around my jaw line. I couldn't believe the difference; after having permanent breakouts on my chin for years, it completely healed after about eight weeks off dairy.

Over the next few years, every time I tried dairy, I had a breakout within 24 hours, like clockwork. I pinpointed that it was cow's milk cream that was the worst offender, which is usually in soups, sauces, and desserts.

After a few years off dairy, I got really serious about healing my gut by eating high-quality food, eliminating processed grains, and incorporating collagen and probiotic supplements. I can now have goat cheese and real Italian Parmigiano-Reggiano (a hard,

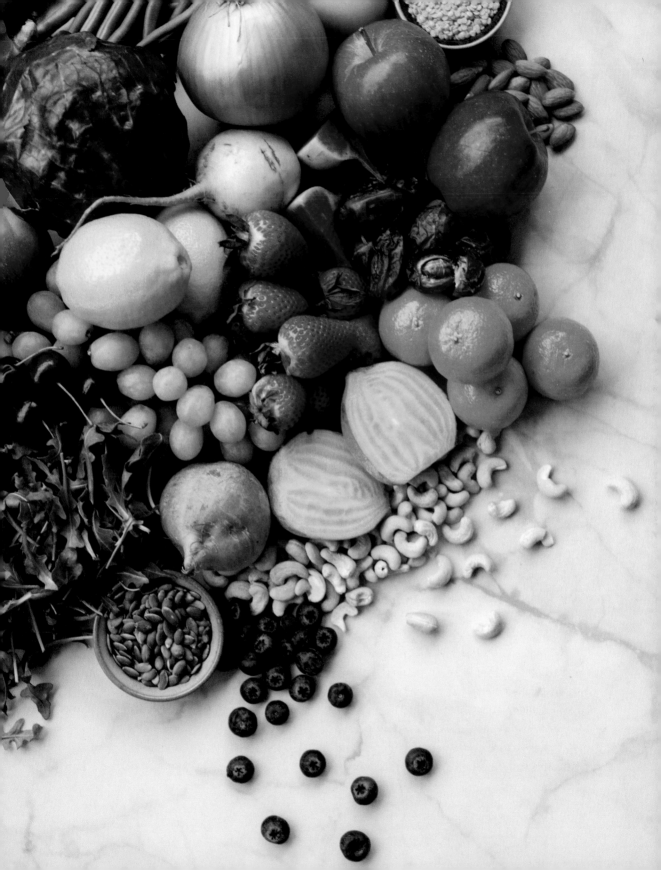

How to Create a Healthy, Bacteria-Friendly Environment in Your Gut

- Follow a low-sugar, high-fiber, real-food eating style: The 28-Day Kick-Start Plan in Chapter 9 will get you started right. Fiber provides the right kind of food for healthy bacteria to flourish, while eliminating added sugars takes away what the bad bacteria like to feed on.

- For the love of all things holy, stop using hand sanitizer and antibacterial wipes, soaps, and toothpastes. They are robbing you—robbing you, I say!—of your good bacteria. Using hand sanitizer while volunteering in a remote village with no running water or toilet paper is one thing. Using it daily because you don't like to touch door handles is another. You need your good bacteria, even on your skin. Don't kill all of it. Wash with hot water and a good old natural soap instead. See Chapter 5 for more information on this.

- Consume naturally fermented foods (see the list on page 54).

- Take a high-quality probiotic supplement on the days when you don't consume naturally fermented food.

- Avoid antibiotics unless absolutely necessary. Overuse of antibiotics can harm the balance of good bacteria in your gut. When they are necessary to fight a bad infection (because sometimes they are), up your intake of probiotics and eliminate all sugars from your diet while on the antibiotic to prevent an overgrowth of the bad bacteria. An antibiotic plus a pint of chocolate ice cream creates a breeding ground for the bad bacteria to take over.

- Stay consistent with your healthy habits. Exercise, quality sleep, and a healthy mindset all contribute to a flourishing gut environment.

long-fermented cheese that is low in cream, not the fake stuff in a plastic shaker bottle) with no issues.

If you suspect you have leaky gut, SIBO, and excess candida or another gut condition, please seek help from a health-care provider. It's perfectly healthy to engage in an elimination diet on your own to gain more self-awareness into what foods heal you (in fact, I included the concept in your 28-day kick-start!), but do

not self-diagnose a medical condition. Lean on an expert for assistance. For now, let's talk about creating a healthy gut microbiome with your daily eating habits.

For optimal gut health, it's crucial to create an inviting place for beneficial bacteria to flourish in your digestive tract, as your gut microbiome can influence your microbiome as a whole. Lactic acid–producing bacteria, such as lactobacillus and bifidobacteria (found in naturally fermented foods and probiotics), will do just that.

You've probably heard of probiotics before, and they're now more crucial than ever. Stress, processed foods, and widely used (but mostly unnecessary) antibacterial agents in everything from hand soap to toothpaste, and the overuse of antibiotics in our modern world may have killed a good amount of your good gut bacteria. So it's great to focus on amping up your good gut bacteria because they can multiply and have a cumulative effect.

Fermented Foods

Naturally fermented foods contain a multitude of friendly bacteria (aka probiotics) that your body needs to thrive. They also add a wonderful, tangy flavor that can take a dish from just okay to *wowza, that's good*. Add some kraut to your salads or mix some coconut yogurt (or Greek yogurt if you tolerate dairy) into your smoothies or overnight oats.

Sorry, even though alcoholic beverages are fermented, they don't count. The alcohol and acids used to ferment the drinks make it nearly impossible for good bacteria to thrive (bummer for us wine lovers, I know).

When I was young, I used to detest sauerkraut. But little did I know, I wasn't eating real sauerkraut. My mom's mom, with steely black hair and Russian roots, was madly in love with her husband, my mom's German dad, thus learned how to make his favorite German dish, called *knoephla*. Knoephla is basically a dumpling made from white flour and milk, sometimes served in soup, sometimes with more potatoes. It's gluten-and-dairy-carb-city,

and as her version didn't contain any spices or flavoring, in my opinion it tasted like flour paste. Even as a kid I knew I didn't like it (I was apparently destined to become a health coach).

My grandmother was a whiz at canning cucumbers with fresh dill, so dinner was usually pickles, knoephla with sauerkraut (another German invention/discovery), and Tang. Remember Tang? That orange drink invented by Germans that became popular in the United States when NASA used it on spaceflights? It was my grandmother's way of showing us that she loved us—Tang did contain vitamin C, along with a whopping 29 grams of sugar per serving. As a result my cousins, my sisters, and I were bouncing off the playset in the backyard while she made the knoephla.

Just like Tang, food companies were starting to make convenience foods and my grandmother's sauerkraut came in a can. Here's what she didn't know: It was just cabbage soaked in vinegar with preservatives made to taste like real sauerkraut.

Real sauerkraut is fermented—lacto-fermented, to be exact—and contains loads of healthy bacteria that keep your gut healthy. Once the canned stuff came out, my grandmother, along with women around the world, stopped making the real versions, both of sauerkraut and other foods. Over the next few decades and into the 1990s, when the low-fat craze hit, the rates of chronic diseases skyrocketed.

It's not my grandmother's or the women (and men) in her generation's fault, it's simply the side effect of overconsuming highly processed food replacements. The good news is

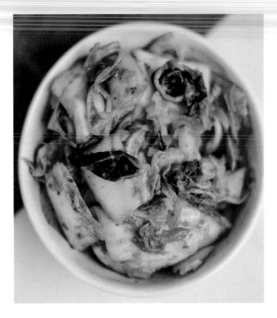

Fermented pickles are making a comeback, which is good news for your gut health—give them a try and enjoy the flavor along with the natural probiotics. Remember, you can find them in the refrigerated section of the grocery store with the other fermented products.

Some examples of naturally fermented foods include:

- Kimchi (Korean-style fermented veggies)

- Real fermented sauerkraut

- Real fermented pickles

- Fermented veggies of any kind, such as pickles made from the lactic acid fermentation process instead of simply being soaked in vinegar

- Raw, unpasteurized apple cider vinegar

- Kefir, either coconut-based or milk-based if you tolerate dairy

- Unsweetened Greek or Icelandic yogurt if you tolerate dairy

- Homemade coconut yogurt, which is great if you're dairy-free (see the recipe for my two-ingredient version on page 188)

- Kombucha tea is fermented but generally doesn't contain high amounts of probiotics, and usually contains added sugar. Choose no-sugar-added kombucha and drink occasionally if desired, but don't rely on it as your main source of probiotics.

that real sauerkraut is actually delicious, inexpensive, and almost ridiculously simple to make yourself at home. You just need cabbage, salt, spices if you want them, a mason jar, and some counter space. You can make it at room temperature and it will keep in your refrigerator for a few weeks.

You can also buy fermented veggies, like sauerkraut or kimchi (sauerkraut's delicious Korean cousin); just remember that the real thing will always be refrigerated at the store. Read the label and make sure they are fermented, not just simply canned in vinegar.

The fermentation process gives foods a naturally tangy bite, which from a culinary perspective adds flavor and interest to your dish while also cutting heavy fatty flavors, which is why you'll usually see some type of pickle on a burger. Real fermented pickles are tangy because of the lacto-fermentation, not simply from being soaked in vinegar like pickles that you find on the shelves of grocery stores.

There are three ways to incorporate a daily probiotic dose into your eating habits:

1. **Purchase fermented foods to add to your food at home.**

    As I mentioned before, real fermented foods are found only in the refrigerated section of your store. Look for raw (unpasteurized) and read about the company before choosing your product. These days, it's easy to find things like fermented "krauts," fermented veggies, or kefir at the grocery store. Like all foods you purchase, be mindful of added sugars and don't heat real fermented foods, as the heat can kill the good bacteria. Enjoy them raw.

2. **Make your own fermented foods at home.**

    The process of lactic acid fermentation turns seemingly plain veggies like cabbage and cucumbers into the aforementioned deliciously tangy and healthful foods like sauerkraut and pickles. Homemade sauerkraut is one of the easiest and cheapest things you can make at home. You can also make your own yogurt at home, or two-ingredient coconut yogurt if you prefer dairy-free like me. (See the recipe on page 188.)

3. **Take a high-quality probiotic supplement.**

    If you find it difficult to incorporate fermented foods into your daily meal plan, or just want extra probiotics, a high-quality probiotic supplement can help. Look for a dairy-free probiotic that contains at least 10 billion to 15 billion colony-forming units (CFUs) at the time of manufacture. That information should be listed on the package.

I eat fermented foods as often as I can, but I'll admit I don't find a way to incorporate them every single day. I do take a probiotic supplement every day when I take my multivitamin.

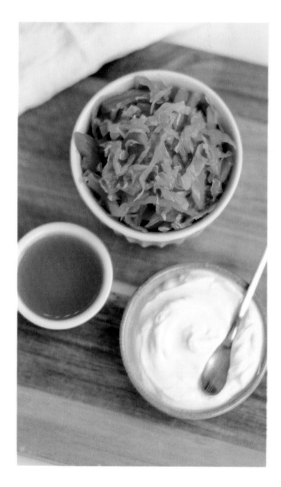

Keeping Your Budget Healthy

Since you and I are pretty good friends by now, let's break taboos and talk about that thing that people aren't supposed to talk about. Don't worry, it's not politics (we don't know each other *that* well), it's money. Specifically, your food budget.

I have friends with very small budgets who spend a lot on food because they value what they put in their mouths, and I have friends with quite a lot of money who spend very little on what they eat because they were raised to believe that food should be as cheap as possible. The opposites are also true: Some people with money spend more because they can, and some people skate by on what they have.

Severe poverty aside, your beliefs and value system set the tone for how you see food and what you spend on it.

I'm not here to tell you what's right or wrong, but I do want to reframe a common belief that eating well has to be expensive. Sure, if you buy grass-fed filet mignon, greens imported from another country, and a lot of packaged yet still heathy convenience food like premade bone broth or cashew butter, then your grocery bill is going to skyrocket.

To maintain a reasonable food budget, buy in-season produce and make most of your own food. In-season produce is usually located at the center or front of the produce section and will vary depending on where you live. Not only does it usually cost less, but it's also the most delicious option in the store, as it was harvested most recently.

Another tip is to use frozen fruits and veggies (read the labels and make sure nothing is added), and shop in bulk bins—and to only buy what you're going to use.

For example, if a recipe calls for one tablespoon of a spice you don't own and you're not sure how much you'll use it, only buy a few tablespoons from the bulk section at your natural grocer instead of an entire jar. Need some pine nuts for a new recipe? Buy the exact amount you need from the bulk section.

Include inexpensive staples like eggs, beans, and lentils in your meal plans, and if you eat meat and fish, ask the meat counter what's the best price that day. Your healthy grocery receipt can be even less than what you spend on all of that highly processed food if you shop smart and buy in season.

Chapter Summary

- There isn't one best way of eating for everyone; you get to choose what eating style works best for you.

- You can choose whether or not you label your eating habits. Based on the moderator/abstainer model, choose to name your eating style (e.g., vegan, paleo) or not based on which way makes you feel more free.

- There is more than one way to lose weight. A few basic truths apply to all of them.

- You don't have to follow a prescribed diet, but you do have to tune into your own body and get back to basics that work. Create an eating style based on the individual nature of the glycemic index, utilize a daily eating window, improve the health of your gut microbiome, choose quality foods, and eliminate the toxic burden of lab-created food additives. All of these basics can fit into any specific diet label should you choose to follow one.

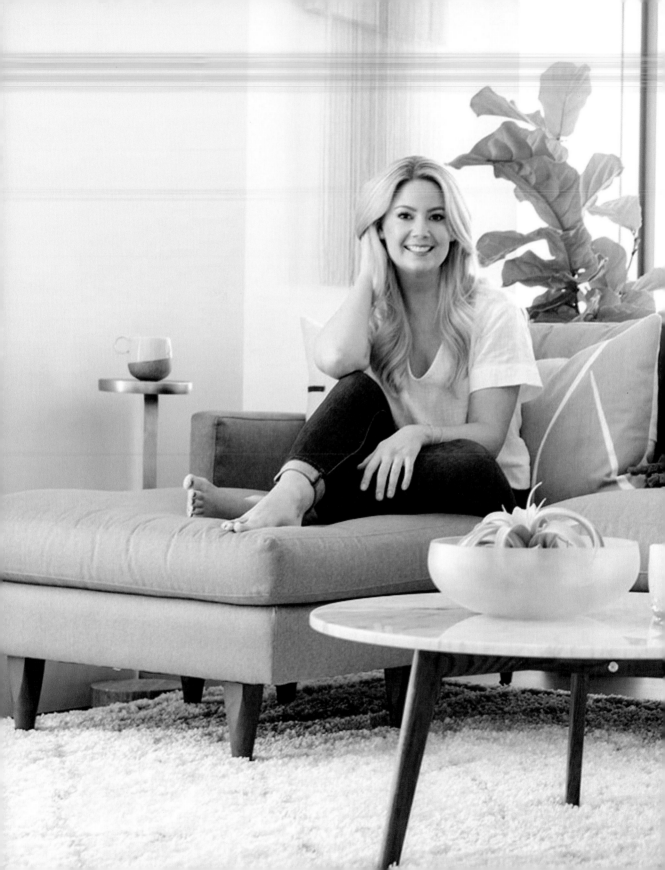

Part II

—

SECRETS OF HEALTHIER LIFESTYLE HABITS

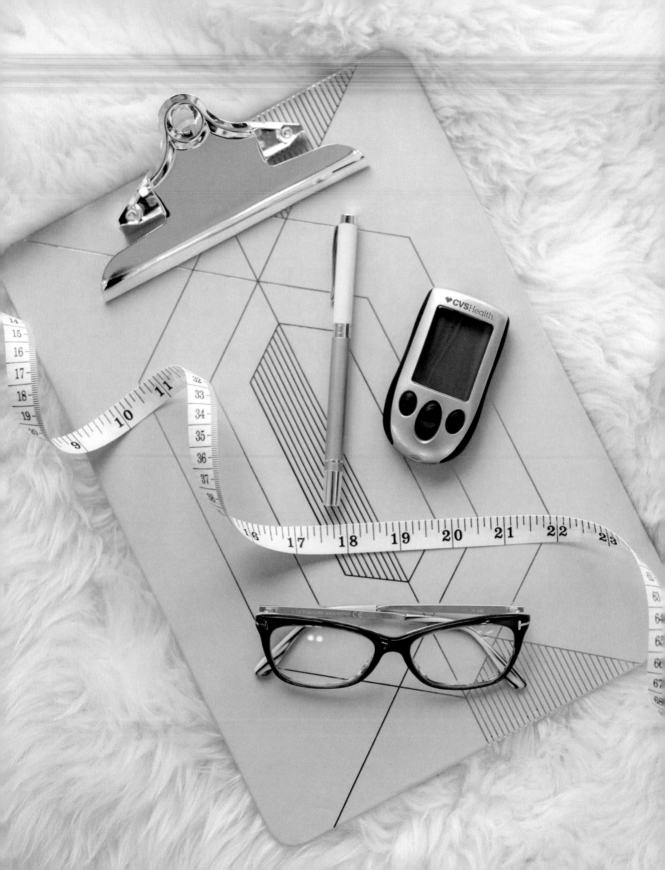

CHAPTER 4

Know Your Numbers

*If you don't know these, getting healthy
may be harder than it needs to be.*

If you've ever made an effort to be healthier but didn't attain the results you were looking for, then you are going to love this chapter. Now that you've got your goals straight and have the tools you need to make healthier food choices, let's talk about another big piece of the health puzzle that most—if not just about all—diets miss.

You might have thought, *Oh great, by numbers she means that I have to count my calories or measure my grams of carbs every day.* Nope! I don't believe that counting calories or weighing your food is healthy over the long term, and may even start the slippery slope to obsession or an eating disorder. That's why this book is all about how to create healthy habits that will serve you for life.

First, we're going to talk numbers. Don't worry—you don't need to be a "numbers person" or do any math. (Side note: My college degree is in math. So if you're a mathlete, too, then we can secretly love math together. For the rest of you, I totally get that most people despise math and I promise never to use the word *mathlete*

again if you promise to keep reading.) When I was doing the research for this book I reviewed a bunch of mainstream diets to remind myself of what was out there. Aside from being bored by seeing the same process over and over simply repackaged with different words, I had an astonishing realization.

Just about every diet I reviewed forgot to mention some critical health numbers that you need to know in order to make progress in your health. It's astonishing because the truth is that no matter how careful and clean you are with what you eat, if the numbers laid out in this chapter are off, then becoming healthier might feel like you're peddling on a stationary bike. You're working pretty hard, but not going anywhere.

After putting thousands of women through online health programs over the years, one of the most common and glaringly obvious desires I've heard from my students is that, while they don't want a diet, they do want structure. Understandably, people don't want to feel deprived and restricted, but they

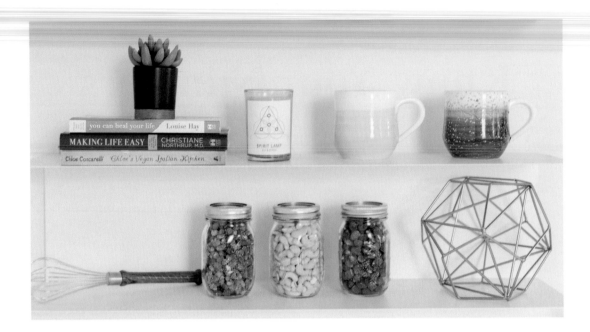

do want a framework of sorts—tools that they can lean on to make better decisions every day. That's the aim of this entire book, and in the space of this chapter I want to lay out some numbers that will do just that.

I'll be the first to admit that none of these numbers are sexy. But do you know what *is* sexy? A woman armed with the knowledge she needs to take control of her own health and her own life. This kind of woman is so sexy that everyone just wants a sexy piece of her. So keep reading, you sexy smartypants.

NUMBERS YOU CAN TRACK YOURSELF

There are important health numbers that you can track and understand yourself, without the help of a health-care professional. When I

ask most women, "What's the most important thing to count when it comes to food?" most say calories. But if counting calories worked, everyone would be at their ideal weight.

You learned in the last chapter why simply reducing calories or starving yourself can lower your metabolism and ultimately not work, so let's talk here about some numbers that *are* useful to count, and how to get into the habit of keeping an eye on them. Mainly, the healthy allowance for grams of added sugar and grams of fiber consumed each day. The good news is that they are both 25, so you only need to remember one number. You don't need to count these things every day for the rest of your life, but you should have a general idea of how much added sugar and fiber is in each of your meals and snacks, so you can create a baseline for yourself.

Tracking Added Sugars

As you remember from Chapter 2, the World Health Organization recommends consuming fewer than 25 grams of added sugar per day—and naturally occurring sugars in whole fruits and veggies don't count in that total. (I consider fruit juice added sugar because it's missing the fiber from the whole piece of fruit.) It adds up fast, so stick to real foods as much as possible to limit added sugars.

To make this super clear, let's look at two seemingly similar examples that aren't so alike after all. I used conservative estimates for these sugar totals, and even then it's shocking. The takeaway? Read labels and watch out for hidden sugar. This is just one more reason to prepare most of your own food, too.

In this example, Scenario 1 looks pretty healthy at first glance, but check out how much sugar is hidden in this daily meal plan. Scenario 2 is just as satisfying and is far better for your health.

MEAL	SCENARIO 1	SCENARIO 2
BREAKFAST	8 ounces of orange juice with nonsugary "whole grain" cereal (25 grams added sugar, 2 grams fiber)	Homemade Hemp & Chia Seed Overnight Oats (see recipe, page 176) with unsweetened almond milk, blueberries, banana slices, and 1 teaspoon of raw honey (6 grams added sugar, 6 grams fiber), with peppermint tea on the side
SNACK	100-calorie snack pack (2 grams added sugar, 1 gram fiber)	1 small apple with unsweetened almond butter (0 grams added sugar, 5 grams fiber)
LUNCH	Entrée restaurant salad with vinaigrette (15 grams added sugar, 6 grams fiber)	Secret-Ingredient Tuna Boats (see recipe, page 230) with avocado (0 grams added sugar, 4 grams fiber)
SNACK	Store-bought nutrition bar (10 grams added sugar, 2 grams fiber)	1 cup Black Bean & Sweet Potato Superfood Salad (see recipe, page 208; 0 grams added sugar, 9 grams fiber)
DINNER	Store-bought marinara over chicken with ½ cup pasta and veggies (12 grams added sugar, 5 grams fiber)	Homemade marinara over chicken with ½ cup quinoa and veggies (2 grams added sugar, 7 grams fiber)
DESSERT	½ cup ice cream (14 grams added sugar)	⅓ cup No-Bake Extra-Chocolatey Chocolate Avocado Mousse (10 grams added sugar, 1 gram fiber)
TOTAL	88 grams of added sugars, 16 grams of fiber	18 grams of added sugars, 32 grams of fiber

As you can see, with a few tweaks, Scenario 2 is much lower in added sugars and has double the fiber. Scenario 2 will set you up for healthy habits, while Scenario 1 will make getting healthy feel much harder than it needs to.

Filling Up on Fiber

Fiber is your body's main way of dumping excess estrogen. I can't stress enough how important this is. Estrogen is one of your main female hormones and you need it, but your body needs to be able to process it and get rid of it, too.

Fiber is estrogen's way out of the body, so pay extra attention to getting enough of it. Not only does fiber help prevent estrogen dominance, it sweeps out your digestive system, de-bloats your belly, and helps you feel full. Consume 25 (and up to 50) grams of fiber per day. Yes, every single day.

Once you get into the habit of this eating plan you won't have to count your grams of fiber—you'll get enough naturally. But if you're just starting out, track your fiber intake to gauge how much you're getting each day.

By nature, fiber comes from carbohydrates. It's the indigestible part of the plant that moves through your digestive system like a spongy broom. There are two types of fiber: soluble fiber that soaks everything up, and insoluble fiber that sweeps it all out.

Don't worry too much about which type of fiber you're getting; if you eat a lot of real food you'll have the right balance naturally.

> # Fiber is your body's main way of dumping excess estrogen.

If you find it challenging to consume your 25 or more grams of fiber per day, consider a good-quality psyllium husk fiber supplement. Stay away from flavored, colored, and most commercial fiber supplements (e.g., ones that rhymes with schmedimucial) as they contain food coloring, added sugars, and other unnecessary chemicals. A natural psyllium-based fiber supplement can be a fantastic addition to your morning shake or overnight oats to help you reach the recommended 25 to 50 grams per day.

We nutritionists like to use the word *elimination* instead of *pooping* because most people find it friendlier. Whatever you call it, you should be doing it at least once per day and it should be natural and easy. If it's runny, you may not be getting enough fiber. If it's hard or in little pellets, you're most likely dehydrated. If you get plugged up, here are two natural remedies that can help: senna tea or magnesium citrate.

Senna is an FDA-approved nonprescription laxative available in teas found at the natural foods store (I like the aptly named Get Regular by Yogi Tea and Smooth Move by Traditional Medicinals). Most people find senna pretty gentle and that drinking the tea at night helps with elimination in the morning. But everyone can react differently, so I suggest taking it for the first time over a weekend or whenever you don't have to be somewhere early the next day.

Another option is magnesium citrate, which works as a natural muscle relaxer (your colon is a muscle) to allow for easier

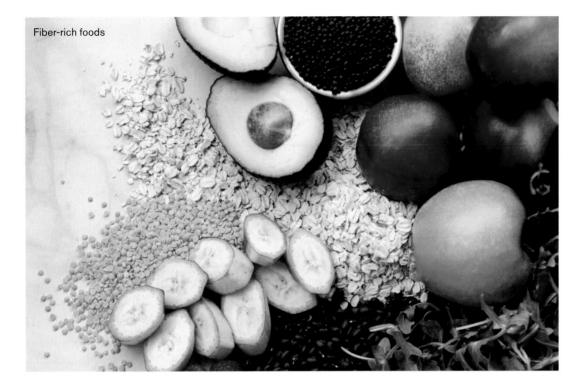

Fiber-rich foods

elimination. Many people like to take this before bed, as the magnesium has a relaxing effect on all of your muscles. Like senna, I suggest taking it for the first time over a weekend when you don't have to be somewhere early the next day.

These natural remedies should be used occasionally when needed and not relied on for everyday elimination. If you feel you need to use them daily, please see a licensed healthcare professional for a consultation.

Drink Like Your Life Depends On It

I consider myself a compassionate and flexible health coach, but the only time I give my clients tough love is when they say, "I just don't like drinking water." Um, do you know what does love drinking water? Your cells.

Your body is almost 60 percent water and every one of your cells needs water to function properly. If you're serious about your health, then drink up. At the very least, the old standby recommendation of eight glasses of water, which is about 64 ounces, will do. Even better, aim to drink half your healthy body weight (in pounds) in ounces each day. So if your natural healthy body weight is 180 pounds, aim for 80 ounces of filtered water each day.

I always recommend filtered water, because the truth is it has to be filtered somewhere. If you don't filter it, your liver has to and it's already your hardest-working organ. Give it a little help by filtering the water ahead, and try to avoid bottled water (most of it is just tap water, and plastic bottles are taking over our oceans). A pitcher-style at-home filter works, or a reverse-osmosis system is even better if it's possible to access one.

Drinking beverages with added or artificial sugars is one of the surest ways for your body to hold on to excess weight and sabotage your Health Habit efforts. By now, most people understand that sugary beverages are trouble, but did you also know that studies have shown that people who use artificial sweeteners (e.g., drink diet soda or use artificial sweetener packets in coffee) actually weigh more than people who don't use them? As I mentioned before, artificial sweeteners can create the same hormonal response in your body as actual sugar. It's best to just avoid them altogether.

Another reason to stay hydrated is that you can mistake thirst for hunger. The same area of your brain signals both. Mild dehydration can mimic hunger as well, leading to overeating when you're really just thirsty. One to two servings of herbal tea (naturally caffeine-free), pure coconut water, or one serving of no-sugar-added kombucha tea are great additions to your daily meal plan if you want something flavorful to sip on.

Tackling the Hard Stuff

Consuming caffeinated beverages such as coffee and green tea is a personal choice. Some people do just fine on a little caffeine . . . and some people don't. If you ever feel jittery or nauseated after a caffeinated beverage it's best to abstain. Too much caffeine can cause adrenal fatigue and disrupt your sleep.

On the flip side, studies show that a little caffeine before a workout can give you a healthy boost in energy for a more effective workout. Nutritionists like myself find it best not to consume caffeine after noon. Always be mindful of your caffeine consumption and when in doubt, take a break.

If you do choose to consume caffeine, limit yourself to one to two small cups per day, and preferably choose organic as you don't wash coffee or tea before consumption. Coffee is the most heavily pesticide-sprayed crop in the world. On the flip side, organic coffee, like green tea, is rich in antioxidants and full of plant nutrients. Black tea also contains caffeine and some nutrients. I personally love coffee and find my mornings are more joyful with it, so I consciously choose to sip my bliss but keep a watch out for caffeine jitters.

Just like caffeine, consuming alcohol is a personal choice. I also love a glass of red wine, but let's not trick ourselves into putting alcohol on a health pedestal. If you don't drink alcohol there's no reason to start. However, a few no-sugar-added alcoholic drinks per week can be part of a healthy eating plan if you lead a generally healthy lifestyle.

If you choose to imbibe occasionally there is some information you should know. Proteins, fats, and carbohydrates have to make it all the way to your small intestine before anything is absorbed into your bloodstream. Water and alcohol, on the other hand, can be absorbed as soon as they reach your stomach. That's why when you consume alcohol on an empty stomach it hits you so quickly.

Alcohol also has to be specifically processed by your liver, which recognizes alcohol

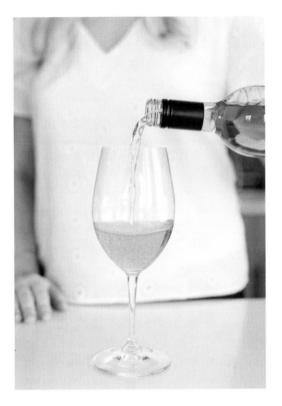

rosés are also dry, depending on the type of grapes used). There are thousands of wines available today, so ask at your local wine store for help.

Beer almost always contains gluten and the carbonation creates bloat fast, so reconsider or use caution when choosing it. And be alert to those sugar-containing mixers added into your cocktails! While liquors like vodka, bourbon, or tequila don't themselves contain added sugars, they can still affect your blood sugar levels and hormones, not to mention your judgment of that late-night pizza delivery service. Remember, anything you add to drinks counts in your 25 grams of added sugars allowance.

Keep up your qualitarian ways, and if you do choose to drink alcohol, choose the best quality you can afford—especially when it comes to wine, because large-scale wine companies add all sorts of additives and sugars to the more inexpensive bottles. And finally, the U.S. dietary guidelines state that women should not consume more than seven alcoholic drinks in a one-week time frame, and never more than three drinks in one 24-hour period.

This information isn't meant to kill your good time—it's meant to keep you healthy enough to enjoy years of good times in good health.

Count Those Daily Steps

While not the steamiest topic in the exercise world, the number of daily steps you rack up matters. Aim for 10,000 to 12,000 steps per day and watch your health improve. Not only will you get a bump in your metabolism, but the increased circulation, muscle movements,

as a poison. As a result, it processes the alcohol first, before any proteins, fats, or carbohydrates. This process can slow your metabolism and hinder fat-burning big time.

In my opinion, excess drinking isn't worth overtasking your liver and slowing down your metabolic processes. If you do consume alcohol, choose wisely. Drier varieties of wine tend to hold less sugar—a glass of high-quality wine contains about 2 grams of sugar, which isn't technically considered an added sugar, but I group it into that category because it doesn't have any nutritional benefits.

Dry varieties of white wine include sauvignon blanc and pinot grigio, and dry varieties of red wine include malbec and syrah (some and energy boost you'll get from hitting this goal all work to improve your health.

Many people also find more connection with others in meeting this goal when they walk with family and friends and schedule social outings around movement. Most smartphones and smart watches have built-in step trackers, or you can find an inexpensive pedometer or fitness tracker, like a Fitbit, to count your daily steps.

Most fitness trackers also have online apps where you can create groups and share your stats. My family is all on an app and my 69-year-old mother beats my two sisters and me just about every single day with her steps— motivation for me to move more! I once saw my sister give her Fitbit to her toddler to run about the kitchen island until her step count caught up with my mom. The hysterical laughter that followed probably made up for the lack of steps that day. (And my sister wants me to tell you that she only did that once.)

Whether it's a morning walk, trail run, lunch stroll, or full-on exercise class, strive to hit this goal every day and to keep moving. Both your mental and physical health will benefit.

Get Intimate with Your Blood Glucose Numbers

This one requires a little more effort, but it is absolutely worth it, because you are worthy of good health. We talked about the glycemic index and how different foods affect different people's blood sugar (blood glucose) levels differently. Now it's time for you to get intimate with your own blood glucose numbers. Even if you are at a healthy weight, these are important numbers to know.

It's well-known that diabetes is an epidemic in the United States. But type 2 diabetes doesn't happen overnight. What you may not realize is that most people who end up with type 2 diabetes live with prediabetes for years, even decades, before being diagnosed.

Diabetes often develops because people have been ignoring their health for years, but knowledge is power, and you can change this trend in your own body. No shame for past decisions. You can consider today day one and change your health. It doesn't matter your weight, age, gender, or background, you need to know these numbers.

First step: Grab a blood glucose monitor at any pharmacy. They are relatively inexpensive—around $30—and often come with a few lancets and strips. The strips are what become more costly, but you'll just need one small pack to get started (you can ask the pharmacist for a generic brand and smallest count of strips and lancets).

Read the instructions to your monitor to learn how to use it. Yes, you'll be pricking your finger for a tiny drop of blood to test, but don't let that scare you off—diabetes is way scarier. Learning to know your blood glucose numbers will not only help you ward off this disease, it may help you control your weight, too.

There are two times of day I want you to measure and record this number: To start, test your fasting blood sugar every morning, right when you wake up, for 10 days straight. Fasting means you haven't had anything to eat or drink except water since going to sleep the night before. Even do it before brushing your teeth, in case your toothpaste has a sweetener in it.

Test at the same time each day, and control your variables (e.g., time of day, fasting state, normal daily happenings) as much as possible. For instance, take into account that if your kid wakes you up at 2 A.M. or you have to wake up at 4:30 A.M. to catch a flight and you have had an abnormal night of sleep, it can affect your morning reading.

Your fasting blood sugar upon waking should be 90 or below. General Western medicine typically says 100 or below, but a modern functional medicine practitioner generally wants to see it at 90 or below. If it is consistently above 90 to 100, then work on reducing your sugar intake and make an appointment with a health-care professional.

The second time to test daily is 30 minutes after you've finished a meal. You can do this after every meal, but do it after at least one (the same meal), again for 10 days straight. Thirty minutes after eating, your blood sugar should remain below 135. If that number is above 135, what you just ate spiked your blood sugar out of the normal range. The next time you eat this food, add some healthy fats and protein to stabilize the effect of the food on your blood glucose levels. Continue to monitor and test this until you know the combination of foods that keeps you in the normal range. These ranges apply to both women and men.

If after 10 days of testing, your fasting and after-meal blood glucose levels are in the normal range, then there's no need to keep testing, at least for now. Make it a habit to repeat this process every six months to a year to know your numbers and keep tabs on yourself. If you're consistently out of the normal range, work on eliminating processed foods, all artificial sweeteners, and excess sugars from your food.

Emotional stress and other health factors can also cause differentials in blood glucose levels. I recommend seeking out a licensed health-care provider for more testing and support if you're consistently out of the normal range, regardless of how you eat.

Nothing is a perfect test or perfect science, so I also want to mention that even if a whole fruit or vegetable on its own spikes your blood sugar, it doesn't mean that it's necessarily bad. You'll benefit from the fiber, natural hydration, vitamins, minerals, and phytonutrients in the food. Just combine it with a healthy protein and/or a healthy fat to keep your blood sugar stable and not miss out on all of nature's benefits. If you combine the fruit with protein and fat and still find yourself out of the normal range, eliminate that fruit and continue to test.

Taking Your Waist Circumference

This is another simple number you can do at home. There is a direct correlation between waist circumference and increased risk of disease.

Now, that's not to say that you can't have a larger waist size and still be healthy. I didn't

> You can consider today day one and change your health.

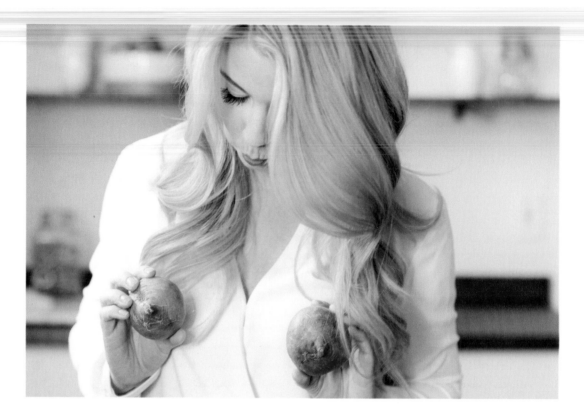

used to recommend knowing this number because, as with weight loss, it's important to remember that you are not a number on a scale or measuring tape. I've shifted to including waist circumference in my program because if knowing it can lead you to choose healthier habits and avoid disease, you should know it.

According to the National Institutes of Health (NIH), a waist circumference of 35 inches/88 centimeters or more in women (40 inches/102 centimeters or more in men) is associated with a higher risk for heart disease and type 2 diabetes.[1]

It's simple to measure your waist. Grab a soft measuring tape (not the one from your toolbox) and stand with your feet a normal hip-width distance apart. Place a tape measure around your middle, just above your hipbones at your natural waist. Measure just after you breathe out. If you're concerned by the result, keep following the steps toward health in this book, and discuss this number with your health-care professional.

Doing Regular Breast Self-Examination

We've all heard this one from the doctor's office, and just about all of us skip it. I'm guilty of that too, but getting familiar with your breast tissue isn't just for your physical health, it also connects you with your feminine spirit, and it's a form of self-care. Plus, 25 percent of breast cancers in the United States are detected by women's self-examination . . . 25 percent![2]

It's totally worth it to take a couple of minutes each month; if you're not sure how, check online—one of my favorites can be found by entering "breast self exam" at mayoclinic.org. This is an important addition to your Health Habit routine.

NUMBERS TO CHECK WITH YOUR DOCTOR

This is where my attorney wants me to remind you that I am not a medical doctor. And trust me, I want to bring that up too because medical doctors—and nurses!—know way more about this than I do, and are your allies in your quest for health.

However, as a health coach and wellness program creator, I've done loads of research into the questions that I get asked when my clients are making their best efforts to reach their health goals but nothing seems to help. What follows are the most common things I ask them to discuss with their health-care professionals. While each of these can seem small, they have a dramatic impact on your well-being if they are out of the normal ranges.

The confusion comes from what's considered "normal." Unfortunately, older standards for optimal ranges are still widely used around the world for some of these tests. The numbers referenced here reflect newer, updated standards that most functional medicine practitioners will follow.

When your lab indicates a value, check it against these updated numbers. For example,

the lab or your doctor might indicate a vitamin D level of 30ng/ml is okay and tell you that you're good to go, but newer standards have set the optimal range at 40 to 65ng/ml. An inexpensive vitamin D_3 supplement is easily absorbed and can raise your levels, and have a big impact on your health.

There are literally hundreds of potential tests your doctor can order and many standard tests that I'm not going to mention here, such as checking your heart rate, blood pressure, and CBC panel. What follows is not a comprehensive checklist, nor is it meant to diagnose a condition. I'm encouraging you to know your numbers as a way to become more aware of your own health.

Work with your health-care provider to determine what tests you need. Here are some to consider:

Test #1:
Vitamin D

Vitamin D is actually a hormone, not just a vitamin, and it plays an important role in your metabolism, immune function, and other vital systems. Symptoms of low vitamin D levels include difficulty losing weight, depression, lethargy, fatigue, getting sick often, muscle pain, and hair loss, among others.

Your glorious body will make enough vitamin D if your arms and legs are exposed to sunlight (without sunblock) for about 15 minutes daily in summer months. When sunlight is absorbed by the skin, your liver and kidneys get the message and turn it into vitamin D—just another reason to thank, and support, your liver for being your hardest-working organ.

You can also get vitamin D from dietary sources, such as fatty fish like salmon, mackerel, or tuna; or from fortified foods including orange juice and cereal. But since we know that cutting out high-glycemic packaged food (like fortified orange juice and cereal) has mega health benefits, they are less desirable options.

Deficiencies arise because you need that exposure or dietary consumption every single day to maintain optimal blood levels. In my experience, it's rare that a client is able to get this much sun exposure and/or eat high-quality fatty fish daily.

Moreover, according to the Harvard Women's Health Watch newsletter, it's virtually impossible to produce enough vitamin D from the sun if you live 37 degrees above the equator (in the United States, that's basically north of Arizona and Tennessee), because the sun doesn't get high enough in the sky for its rays to penetrate the atmosphere.[3]

Optimal blood levels of vitamin D are between 40 and 65ng/mL (or 100 to 160 nmol/L for those of you who use the metric system). If you are low, take a vitamin D_3 supplement and retest in three months. I take a 2,000 IU tablet of vitamin D every day, even in summer, and my vitamin D levels hover right around 65ng/ml year-round. Everyone will be different, just get tested and add a supplement as needed.

Test #2:
Thyroid-Stimulating Hormone (TSH)

In laymen's terms, thyroid-stimulating hormone (TSH) is secreted by your pituitary gland; its job is to tell your thyroid gland to secrete the right amount of thyroid hormones. Your thyroid plays a critical role in your metabolic processes as well as just about every system in your body.

If your TSH is normal, that means your body is making enough thyroid hormones. If your TSH is high, on the other hand, it means your pituitary gland is trying to stimulate more thyroid hormone production but it might not be working.

So high TSH indicates low thyroid levels. This condition is known as hypothyroidism, and symptoms include but are not limited to fatigue, weight gain, often feeling cold, hair loss, and dry skin.

More than 12 percent of the U.S. population will develop a thyroid condition in their lifetime, and women are five to eight times more likely than men to have thyroid problems. Up to 60 percent of those with thyroid disease are unaware of their condition,[4] so it's important to get your TSH checked if you often have low energy levels or find it difficult to lose weight. Many labs and doctors use older standards of "normal" TSH levels between 0.3 and 5.0 mU/L. According to my own functional medicine practitioner, 5.0 is far too high.

I've been treated for my own low thyroid condition since age 18 and all of my doctors—along with most endocrinologists—agree that a TSH as close to 1.0 is ideal. I've been working with doctors for years to get to the root cause of why my thyroid levels are so low, and I wish I had an answer for you (perhaps in a future book!).

The fundamental reasons for low thyroid levels remain mostly a mystery, but new ideas emerge every day. Treating the root cause is always the main goal of a functional medicine practitioner, but even when this remains unknown, it's still important to manage the condition. I manage my low thyroid levels by taking a T4 hormone replacement (known generically as levothyroxine) each morning. Although levothyroxine is a synthetic, it is bio-identical to the T4 (thyroid hormone) produced in your body.

There are also animal-derived thyroid replacements, called glandulars, that some people find more "natural." These are derived from pigs, purified, and are not bio-identical to your hormones. I took a glandular for a while and my condition became worse, but you may have a different experience.

All in all, I feel great since learning to manage my thyroid levels and I continue to monitor them closely. If I'm not sleeping well, if I'm gaining weight, or if I feel off in general when nothing else has changed it's the first thing I check.

The important thing is to be in charge of your own health and work with your health-care provider to find the best solution for you. There's no shame in taking a little help from Western medicine while you continue to explore the root cause of an ailment.

I could go on and on, but I'll finish my thyroid rant by letting you know that there are multiple thyroid hormones and tests, and your doctor may choose to do a full thyroid panel to determine what is happening with you, which I also recommend. Explore that with your health-care provider as needed.

> **The important thing is to be in charge of your own health.**

Test #3: Cortisol

Cortisol is your main stress hormone; it's made by your adrenal glands and released naturally in your body each day. It affects your energy levels by regulating the release of glucose and maintaining normal awake periods.

Maintaining normal cortisol levels is critical to maintaining a healthy weight and healthy sleep cycles. Normal cortisol levels start out lower in the morning, gently peak early in the day, then naturally fall as evening sets in.

All lab tests are a snapshot in time, and this is especially important to consider when testing cortisol. A specifically stressful event or day can send this snapshot out of whack. However, having your cortisol tested can give you an idea if your levels are in the normal range. Some doctors will just test morning cortisol, and some will do four tests in the same day to make sure your levels rise and fall within normal ranges. I prefer the four tests in the same day if feasible.

You may not even need a lab test to know if your cortisol levels are abnormal—chronic levels of physical or emotional stress, inconsistent sleep cycles, or having erratic or dragging energy are all signs of abnormal cortisol levels. If you have that "wired but tired" feeling of not being able to fall asleep, you may have abnormal cortisol levels.

This is one area for which stress reduction is really the only antidote—you can't cheat your way to normal cortisol levels with food or supplements in the long term. Even if you're eating well, exercising, and doing everything "right," excessive amounts of stress can dramatically affect cortisol levels, which in turn affect your body, weight, and sleep.

I had my annual physical with my functional medical practitioner right after signing the deal for this book. At the time, life was great. Hectic, yes. But overall, business was great, relationships were steady, and I had a sense of excitement about life. I was having a hard time falling asleep and feeling a little tired, but those things had been my norm since I was a teenager so I didn't think much of it.

At my physical, my doctor said, "Well, the good news is that your thyroid is right on point. The bad news is that your cortisol is too low in the morning and too high at night." I said, "That's strange, life is so good right now!" She knew I had just signed the book deal, and replied, "Liz, your body can't differentiate 'good' or 'bad' stress. It doesn't know if you're running from a tiger [bad unless you are a tiger], or feeling the massive stress of writing your first book [good if you are a blogger who wants a book deal]. Stress is stress—it doesn't matter where it comes from."

She prescribed that I do more stress-reducing activities like sitting still while breathing or meditating and low-impact movement like yoga. She also suggested that I try an adaptogenic herb called ashwaganda in the evenings, but the stress-reducing activities were the biggest piece of the puzzle. I had my cortisol levels back to normal within a few months. (See page 32 for more on adaptogenic herbs.)

Test #4: A1C

We've already discussed how you can check your blood glucose levels at home. An A1C test (also called hemoglobin A1C) is performed by your doctor and reflects your average blood glucose levels over the prior three months.

You might be wondering, *Why check at the doc if I'm testing at home?* It's because I don't think you can be too aware of these numbers, and some doctors won't even test for this until you're well on your way to diabetes. As Benjamin Franklin once wrote, "An ounce of prevention is worth a pound of cure." Even if you are seemingly healthy, ask your doctor to add this test to your lab order. It's another inexpensive test to help you see the picture of your overall health.

ANNUAL WELL-WOMAN EXAM

While not necessarily a number, an annual exam remains important for catching things early. I've noticed a trend among my clients to skip their preventative Western medicine checkups once they've ventured deep into other areas of wellness and alternative medicine.

Now, don't get me wrong, I'm all about the healing powers of your own body, using food as medicine, and exploring natural and ancient healing modalities. I've meditated, chanted at retreats in the woods, and participated in Mayan cacao ceremonies in the jungle (which prompted a childhood friend who saw the photo to text my sister and ask if I was okay; little did she know that yes, I was entirely okay and even had a little bit of a natural high from

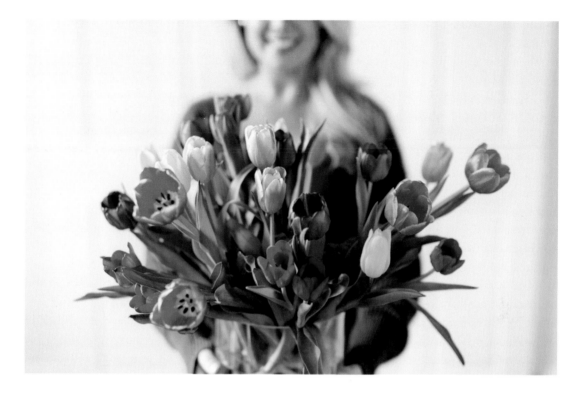

the fresh cacao—raw chocolate, totally safe).

I've also done things for the sake of wellness that I can't mention here because my dad is going to read this book. For all intents and purposes, I'm an alternative-medicine-loving hippie devoted to my inner spiritual goddess, and I have a feeling you have a little alternative-medicine-loving hippie in you, too. But that doesn't excuse either of us from not being informed about our physical health in the here and now.

According to the World Health Organization, cervical cancer is the second-most common type of cancer among women. Cervical cancer is considered preventable because it has a long preinvasive state, there are screening programs available (e.g., a Pap smear or visual inspection), and treatment of preinvasive lesions is effective.[5]

Your annual well-woman exam is often covered as preventative medicine at no cost under insurance, and some providers will even combine all the tests discussed in this chapter into one appointment. Remember when we talked about goals in the first chapter? A great goal this week would be to call and schedule your next well-woman exam.

AUTOIMMUNE SYMPTOM CHECK

This isn't so much a number, but rather a topic to explore with your health-care provider if you have mystery symptoms such as fatigue, weight gain, excessive bloating or digestive issues, skin issues, pain, hair loss, insomnia, or anything else going on with your health that you can't explain.

Approximately one in five Americans—that's 50 million people in the United States alone—suffer from autoimmune diseases.[6] Women are more likely than men to be affected by an autoimmune condition, and if one goes undiagnosed or untreated, getting healthier might feel a lot harder than it needs to.

There are multiple theories as to what causes autoimmune diseases and why they may be on the rise. My best advice is to not spiral out of control down the Internet rabbit hole of information, but rather to arm yourself with as much information as possible and keep working with your health-care provider.

Autoimmune conditions can be tricky to diagnose, so try new ways of eating or treatments as necessary. I was diagnosed with Hashimoto's thyroiditis because my thyroid antibodies were slightly high, but as they were never high again I believe mine to be a misdiagnosis.

New science suggests that chronic infections can also present as autoimmune symptoms, which is what happened to me. My misdiagnosis led me down a new path of exploring the possibility of reactivated Epstein-Barr virus (EBV), which later tests would reveal I do have.

If you have mystery symptoms, I suggest asking your doctor to add both an active EBV test and Lyme disease test with your other blood work so you can understand if your body is fighting a chronic infection. There isn't a standard treatment for dealing with EBV, Lyme, or most chronic infections, but at least you'll know what's happening in your body. Mold toxins, known as mycotoxins, can also contribute to mystery symptoms. Living a healthy lifestyle (and eliminating mold toxins if they are causing trouble) can help you feel better while you explore the root cause of your symptoms.

I know how frustrating mystery symptoms can be. It may be an autoimmune condition, chronic viral infection, or mycotoxin invasion, or it may not be. Regardless, you are not crazy and I believe you. If you have unexplained symptoms and a conventional doctor tells you that you're fine, keep advocating for your own health. Seek out the help of a naturopath or functional medicine specialist and don't give up. Only you live in your body and you are always your own best health advocate.

WHAT ABOUT CHOLESTEROL?

The tremendous amount of negative media about high cholesterol in the 1980s and 1990s scared many people into thinking that testing for this was critical. But as science and medicine have evolved, it's now understood that cholesterol is necessary for healthy brain function. In fact, 25 percent of the cholesterol in the body is found in the brain. It's also a building block for vitamin D, hormones, cell membranes, and bile acids used in digestion.

All that to say, cholesterol's pretty freaking important and suppressing it with drugs can harm every system in your body. Moreover, dietary cholesterol (for example, the cholesterol in an egg) does not necessarily impact blood cholesterol (interesting, I know).

Most modern functional medicine specialists don't fret if your cholesterol is slightly elevated. In fact, they would rather see higher blood cholesterol than put you on a statin drug (a type of drug that lowers blood cholesterol) because your brain and cells need it. With regard to life expectancy and heart disease, it's also interesting to note that people with high cholesterol tend to live longer, and that people with heart disease are more likely to have low levels of cholesterol.

Like all numbers here, work with your health-care provider. If they suggest a statin drug, I urge you to read *Statin Nation* by Justin Smith. Do your own research, including reading information outside of the drug manufacturer's literature. It's still your choice to take it, but you'll at least have the information you need to know what it's doing to your body. I'm all for Western medicine, but in my opinion statins might be the worst drugs ever approved for human consumption.

Chapter Summary

- Consume no more than 25 grams of added sugars per day.

- Consume at least 25 grams of fiber each day.

- Consume half your body weight (in pounds) in ounces of filtered water each day.

- Take 10,000 steps each day (or exercise equivalent).

- Get familiar with your blood glucose levels and know your waist circumference.

- Don't skip your monthly breast self-exam.

- Make an appointment now for your annual physical, and consider requesting the tests to know the numbers outlined in this chapter.

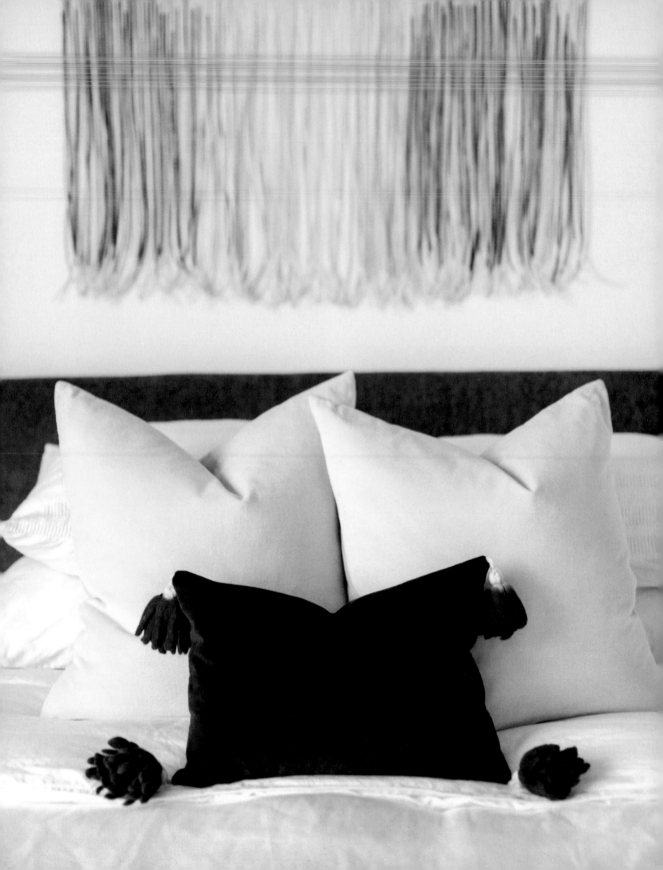

CHAPTER 5

Detox Your Environment

Your internal environment is deeply linked
to your external environment.

Your health is so much more than what you eat. Sure, what you eat matters. The food you put in your mouth makes up the building blocks of your cells, which form not only your bones, tissue, and organs but also your hormones, the chemical pathways your brain uses to communicate, and all the other magic that keeps your body running.

You already know that what you eat influences your health, but did you know that the habits that govern how you operate in other areas of life, like how you create (or disregard) your home environment, and the routines you consciously (or unconsciously) follow each day, also dramatically affect your health?

These non-food factors are just as important as what you put in your mouth. In fact, your non-food lifestyle factors—from how you keep your home space, to how you set up your days, to whom you choose to interact with and how—are what create the mindset and subconscious cues that make you want to take better care of yourself.

Your internal environment is deeply linked to your external environment. Don't worry, I'm not going to tell you to meditate for six hours a day or go do a self-help seminar (although those things can be great!). But I *am* going to ask you to take a good hard look at becoming more conscious about your environment and mindset, because how you spend your days is how you live your life.

Sure, milestones are important and should be celebrated. But the bulk of your life is lived in your daily routines and habits, which can be both healthy and enjoyable. If you don't intentionally get in the habit of crafting a healthy home environment, healthy self-care routines, and healthy boundaries with other people's actions and emotions, you might spend your days spinning your wheels or feeling stuck. And by stuck I mean that you know how to be healthier, you're just not doing it. It's time to pay attention to developing these habits.

SPEAKING FROM EXPERIENCE

A few years ago I sold my gorgeous 2,300-square-foot home, all of my leather and wood furniture, and donated more than half of my possessions to friends and various charities. All in all, I estimated that I got rid of about 85 percent of what I had owned in one fell swoop.

Now, this is an extreme case, and I don't expect everyone do to it. It was a specific season of life for me. I had gone through a painful divorce a few years prior and took time for healing with local friends and family. Life became stable again, and I felt better than I'd ever felt before. I started to crave travel and more exploration.

Selling the house and furnishings was a no-brainer because I lived in a highly desirable area, didn't know how long I wanted to roam, and the furniture was very big and specific to the lodge-y look of my Montana home. It made financial sense to sell instead of paying to store it (because, spoiler alert: How consciously you eat, how consciously you set up your home, and how consciously you care for your finances are all probably pretty similar).

I reveled in efficiency mode. I didn't own a lot, and I didn't have any recurring household bills anymore. I took my lightened self on a trip around the world, spending the fall in New York City with business friends, part of the winter in Central America on a dance and yoga retreat, then alone to the beach to write, back home for the holidays, then a month in Bali masterminding with business friends and indulging in daily $5 spa treatments.

Without my even intending it, a light, airy sense of wholeness extended into every facet of my life. I made quick new friends to laugh with and had long, soul-filling conversations with old ones. I talked to my sisters and parents almost every day, and had so much social time that I barely even spent one evening alone. I ate mostly vegan and walked almost six miles every day. My business flourished and my bank account grew. It was a glorious half year.

Before I took that leap, though, I was scared. I thought all of my "stuff" was useful and necessary. I had a happy life. My home was nice and I was comfortable there. I was close to family and friends. But once I worked up the courage to listen to that little voice inside my head telling me to play bigger and change my environment, I had the happiest, healthiest year of my life.

I knew that there was a connection between home and health, but I had no idea how much my physical space was influencing my habits or overall health.

Eventually, I felt the need to ground myself back into my own space. I found a permanent (for now) home and replenished what I needed. When it comes to decluttering, there are a variety of great resources and books (hi, Marie Kondo!) about decluttering your home and physical spaces. I highly recommend lightening up this way.

In this book—in the spirit of making a Health Habit you'll keep—we're going to talk

> How you spend your days is how you live your life.

more about how to set yourself up for success by creating morning and evening routines that allow you to thrive. So yes, do the de-cluttering. Here, I'm going to teach you how to look at the non-food factors that influence your health to help your healthy habits flow in harmony.

Never underestimate the power of your physical environment. It has been understood for centuries in systems such as feng shui that the space you inhabit influences your mood, thoughts, emotions, and habits.

Clutter and mess in your physical space creates clutter and mess in your mind. While you don't have to go full minimalist, it's important to keep the energy in your physical space open, harmonized, and de-chemicalized as much as possible. Your physical environment is one of the single biggest factors of whether or not you will achieve your health goals.

The right environment can make you more efficient, focused, and—perhaps most important—consistent. Environmental cues trigger certain behaviors, for better or worse. A hot-water kettle and beautiful bowl filled with herbal tea waiting to be brewed that has a permanent spot on your counter will result in a hot cup of tea when you crave something comforting, while store-bought jumbo muffins filled with sugar, white flour, and chemical preservatives in the same spot will also fill that need, with different effects on your health. Likewise, a pantry filled with expired food and nutritionally void chips and cookies will cue you to order takeout when you're in need of a quick meal.

YOUR BODY WILL THANK YOU

Your healthy—or unhealthy—habits build on each other. When you clean up the way you eat, you'll naturally influence other habits in your daily life. Once you start reading the labels on food, you will naturally progress to reading the labels on things like laundry detergent, or vice versa.

Not only does detoxing your home environment alleviate mental clutter, but it also rids your home of physical toxins. Toxic ingredients in beauty products and cleaning products can disrupt your hormones and sabotage your health.

You might be thinking, *Is it really true that ingredients in beauty products can harm me? I mean, aren't those vetted and monitored by the government?* But the government only worries about the safety of products after something has an issue; there's no formal process or audit to bring beauty and cleaning supplies to the market. It's up to you to get into the habit of paying attention to what you use on your body and in your home.

What you apply to your skin or come in contact with in your environment can sink into your skin and enter your bloodstream. Some ingredients smoothed onto your skin will even show up in a urine test. Your lymphatic system, liver, kidneys, and other organs are tasked with processing these harmful ingredients out of your

> Environmental cues trigger certain behaviors, for better or worse.

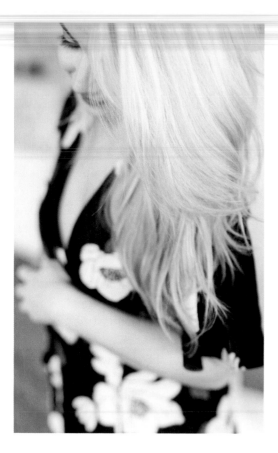

Weight gain, acne, fatigue, depression, and irregular menstrual cycles (not to mention fertility issues) can all be caused by xenoestrogens and other hormone disruptors. That means the real culprit of your low energy or inability to lose weight could be the toxic ingredients in your beauty and cleaning routines.

Since there are hundreds of chemical additives legally available—and new ones popping up every day—it's almost impossible to create a list of everything to avoid. In general, stay away from any products with the following: parabens, triclosan, butylated ingredients (BHA), formaldehyde-releasing ingredients, phthalates, or polytetrafluoroethylene (PTFE), also known as Teflon. You don't have to do all of these things at once if it feels too overwhelming. But to improve your health, and the health of your family, take the time to work through these sections and move toward detoxing your home and environment. Let your healthy habits build on themselves over time and spread into other areas of your life.

THE KITCHEN

First up, the kitchen, command center for your health. What you keep around, how you pay attention to it, and the care and love you feel in your kitchen all affect your physical health. Creating a space you love—one you look forward to spending time in—will draw you to it, making home cooking more enjoyable.

Since I don't live with you and neither one of us is looking for a new roommate, I don't know your cooking habits and what you love to eat. I hope that you cook at home often and

body but, depending on how efficient your body is, those toxins can cause problems.

Some of the chemicals in beauty products are considered endocrine disruptors, aka hormone disruptors. Some of them can even act *as* hormones, specifically estrogens. These are called "xenoestrogens" and can cause a whole lot of mess in your body. Using a bunch of toxic chemicals in skincare or cleaning supplies can be similar to pumping your body full of a whole bunch of extra estrogen, which can throw off all of your other hormones and make getting healthy even harder.

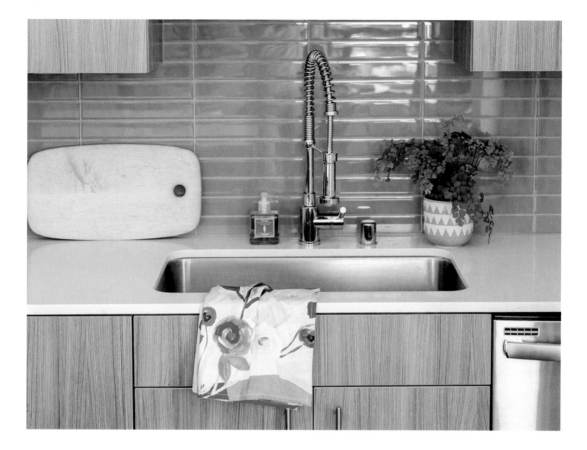

eat healthy food (and if you don't, go back and read Chapters 2 and 3 again).

I'm not going to give you a big long list of what to keep around or things you need to buy. (Nothing makes me crazier than a bag of decomposed produce that was pushed to the back of the fridge to rot.) Instead, I'll give you a few suggestions and then you can customize your space from there.

I tend to think it's better to have a lean, less-is-more kitchen philosophy. You don't need special herb cutters (they're just little scissors! What a racket.), 18 different zesters (one grater for everything is enough for the citrus, garlic, ginger, hard cheeses, and anything else you need to grate finely), or a small appliance for every type of dish out there (I'm looking at you, bread-maker taking up half the counter).

To prevent overwhelm, before you bring something into your kitchen ask yourself, *Do I already have something that can do what this does?* That's a great rule to apply to your entire life. Special ceramic pizza cutter? Nah, my sharp chef's knife will do that. Fancy spiral apple-peeling gadget? Sounds fun, but my $3 veggie peeler does the same thing. New boyfriend who wants my Netflix password? Nope, I've already got four family members for that.

TOOLS THAT BELONG IN A HEALTHY KITCHEN:

A good cutting board that you replace often and as soon as it appears to be worn out

A sharp chef's knife (for the love of all things holy, get your knives sharpened)

Nonreactive cooking utensils made from wood, bamboo, stainless steel, and/or silicone

An all-purpose mixing bowl that can double as a serving and storage bowl (a big glass one with a lid is great)

A Dutch oven is extremely versatile (this is an enamel-covered cast-iron pot that has many uses and can be used on the stove top or in the oven)

A stainless-steel, ceramic, or cast-iron sauté pan (Teflon/PTFE-free)

Glass storage containers, like mason jars, Pyrex, or other glass containers with lids

Bakeware made from ceramic, enamel-covered cast iron, tempered glass, or stoneware

A high-speed blender is a healthy cook's best friend

Non-toxic cleaning supplies (see page 87 for ideas)

TOOLS THAT DO NOT BELONG IN A HEALTHY KITCHEN:

Nonstick pans coated with Teflon and PTFE. I know, getting rid of nonstick pans is a huge inconvenience, but those nonstick chemicals have been banned by the Environmental Protection Agency (EPA) and the replacement ones aren't any better. Cook in stainless-steel, ceramic with a spray of healthy oil, cast-iron, or enamel-covered cast-iron pans.

Plastic cutting boards, plastic utensils (hey, melted spatula), and plastic storage containers all have to go. Not only are they ruining our environment, they are ruining your health. And don't think that BPA-free plastic is any better. Companies just replace the BPA with something just as harmful. Use glass or parchment paper storage instead.

Plastic or melamine plates and drinking cups. You guessed it—these leach chemicals into your food. Melamine kitchenware is a combo of melamine and formaldehyde, also known as melamine resin. It's only considered safe if it doesn't get hot. I think it's best to not use it.

One-time-use plastics, like plastic straws and bags. Try to at least limit these as much as possible; they are bad for your health and horrible for our environment. Parchment or beeswax paper, cloth or washable silicone bags, or glass containers can make a great replacement for plastic bags.

Things you don't use anymore. If you haven't used it in a year, get rid of it to create space for something that inspires you, or leave that spot empty and enjoy more feelings of spaciousness.

THE LAUNDRY

Oh laundry, you're one thing I just want someone else to do for me. But alas, until someone invents magic robots to wash, dry, and fold perfectly, we're just going to have to do it ourselves.

While I can't make doing your laundry any easier, I can help you make it healthier. Here's the rub: We spend nearly a third of our lives sleeping in our sheets. That doesn't even include all the great sex I hope you're having that sometimes happens in your bed. But it's the sheets I'm talking about, so stay with me.

You know that freshly washed scent of your sheets? Well, that scent is not as clean as you think. In fact, it's not clean at all. Remember when I told you that food companies spend big bucks to create flavors that keep you addicted to food? Well, manufacturing companies do something similar with scent and color additives to make you think you're using the best detergent.

But the blue color and fake breezy scents aren't worth it. One study showed that air vented from dryers from clothes washed in top-selling scented liquid laundry detergent contains 25 hazardous chemicals, including two that are classified as carcinogens. Yikes. This happens during *each* cycle. Double yikes!

Look for laundry detergents free of artificial dyes and fragrances, and avoid fabric softeners and dryer sheets. A half cup of distilled white vinegar in the wash will do the same job

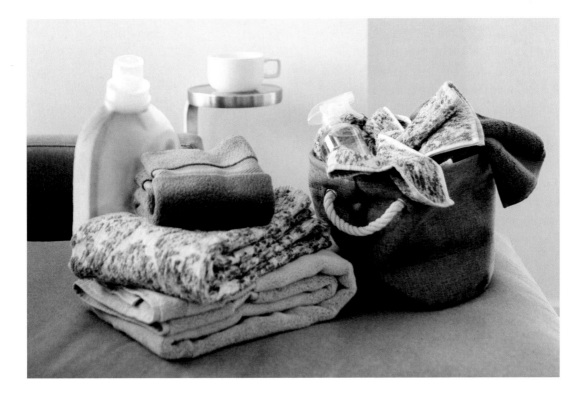

as a fabric softener, and wool or silicone dryer balls can eliminate static without the nasty chemicals.

There are also dozens of natural laundry detergents on the market; it's best to read the company's mission statement and do your own research to choose one. From my personal experience, they've come a long way in being gentler on clothes. At the very least, wash your jammies, underwear, sheets, and towels in a natural detergent to decrease your chemical exposure.

CLEANING SUPPLIES

Just like the laundry, the rest of your cleaning supplies might be bringing harmful chemicals into your home unnecessarily. As with food, read the labels—if you can't pronounce the ingredients, they're probably not natural.

Do your research and buy from brands you trust. Or, make your own natural and inexpensive cleaning supplies at home from OG cleaners such as distilled white vinegar and baking soda. Distilled white vinegar is a natural disinfectant, and baking soda is a way to add grit to natural cleaning sprays (for hard to clean spots). Distilled white vinegar can also decalcify clogged shower heads and faucets. I like to add essential oils to my cleaning spray for a delightful scent (and tend to go a little heavy), so add your favorites and adjust the amounts per your preferences.

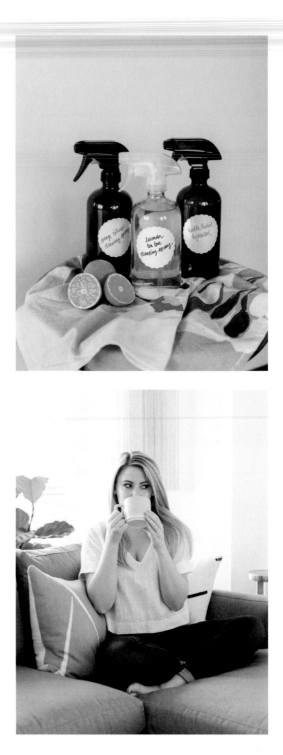

HEALTHY DIY HOME CLEANERS AND SPRAYS

HEALTHY FLOOR CLEANER	Mix a solution of ½ cup distilled white vinegar to ½ gallon of warm water.
HEALTHY COUNTER SPRAY	Mix one part distilled white vinegar to one or two parts filtered water (the more vinegar, the stronger it is) in a spray bottle. **Optional:** add ½ tablespoon of baking soda to give the spray grit for hard-to-clean spots. **Optional and recommended:** add 10 to 20 drops of your favorite essential oils for a pleasant spelling spray.
GREEN GLASS CLEANER	Mix equal parts of distilled white vinegar and water. Elizabeth's mom's trick: use black-and-white newsprint on the glass instead of a towel for lint-free cleaning. (It's strange, but it works!)
TO CLEAN THE DISHWASHER	Place 2 cups distilled white vinegar in a glass bowl on the bottom rack of an empty dishwasher. Run a full cycle (no dishes, no soap added). Wipe the inside edges and door with a towel sprayed with the healthy counter spray above once the cycle ends.
DECALCIFY YOUR SHOWER HEADS AND FAUCETS	Soak the clogged-up hardware, such as your shower head, overnight in a bowl of undiluted distilled white vinegar; it will run clean in the morning.
HEALTH HABIT HYDROSOL	A hydrosol is all all-purpose spray, use it as a room spray, linen spray, or even body spray. Here is my favorite: In a 16 ounce glass spray bottle, combine two cups filtered water with 1 tablespoon witch hazel. Add 10 drops of lavender, 8 drops of frankincense, and 5 drops of orange or lemon essential oils. (I love this scent combo, but feel free to mix up the combination to make it your own.) Shake well before each use.
HEALTH HABIT BED LINEN SPRAY	In a 16 ounce glass spray bottle, combine two cups filtered water with two tablespoons witch hazel. Add 15 drops of lavender, 10 drops of rose, and 6 drops of frankincense essential oils. Spray a gentle mist onto your bed linens or bath towels each night before bed. Shake well before each use. (This makes a wonderful homemade housewarming gift as well.)
CITRUS EUCALYPTUS CLEANING SPRAY	In a 16-ounce glass spray bottle, combine one cup distilled white vinegar with one and a half cups filtered water. Add 15 drops of orange, 10 drops of lemon, and 10 drops of eucalyptus essential oils.
LAVENDER TEA TREE CLEANING SPRAY	In a 16-ounce glass spray bottle, combine one cup distilled white vinegar with one and a half cups filtered water. Add 12 drops of lavender, 10 drops tea tree essential oils. Adjust oils as needed to your preference.

BEAUTY PRODUCTS

When you start along a healthier path with your food, the label reading and inclination toward more natural products will (hopefully) move into your beauty routine, too.

According to the Environmental Working Group, the average U.S. woman uses 12 personal-care products and/or cosmetics a day, containing 168 different chemicals.[1] It's estimated that there are more than 13,000 chemicals used in beauty products, and only about 10 percent of them have been studied for safety. Moreover, the FDA does not require approval for personal-care products. Instead, companies are on the honor system for substantiating the safety of their goods. Since there are literally too many chemicals added to beauty products to cover in one book, my best advice is to do your research and buy from brands you trust.

Your beauty product routine covers everything from what you put on your hair and skin, to what you use to brush your teeth and care for your nails. It's a big category, but there is one ingredient I specifically want to point out.

I mentioned triclosan back in Chapter 3, when we covered your gut microbiome. Triclosan is an antibacterial agent found in hand sanitizer, hand soaps, toothpaste, and other antibacterial products. It's been linked to low thyroid function and an imbalance of good gut bacteria. Although the FDA banned the use of triclosan in hand soaps and body wash in 2016 because of its harmful effects, it's still widely used in other products. If anything, do not use toothpaste with triclosan as it can go directly into your digestive system and kill your good bacteria.

When I think about my overall microbiome and the necessity of good bacteria, I always think of a story that my friend and world-renowned OB-GYN Dr. Christiane Northrup told me over lunch. She was reminiscing about her early days as a doctor delivering babies, and how surgical birth prep had become. Women had been giving birth in every environment imaginable since the dawn of time, yet here she was in the 1980s, required to shave women completely for "sanitary" purposes and sterilize everything in sight.

During one delivery, the mother wanted her baby put on her chest immediately. At the time this natural and common postdelivery bonding experience was not practiced because of the fear of germs. When Dr. Northrup followed her wishes and placed the baby on her mother, immediately upon arrival a colleague exclaimed, "You can't do that! It's not sterile!" To which she replied, "That baby just came out of the birth canal—if you want it to be sterilized you're going to have to boil it!" He looked at her, aghast at the descriptive statement. She looked at him, aghast for wanting to take away all of the child and mother's good bacteria. I'm always grateful for this story—it's a good reminder not to let people or things rob us of our good bacteria.

Again, do your research when it comes to beauty and personal-care products, and buy from brands you trust. Your skin is your largest organ, and one of your detox organs to boot. When harmful chemicals are absorbed through it, they not only hinder your skin's ability to detox (toxins are supposed to be coming out through the skin via sweat, not in via products), your liver, lymphatic system,

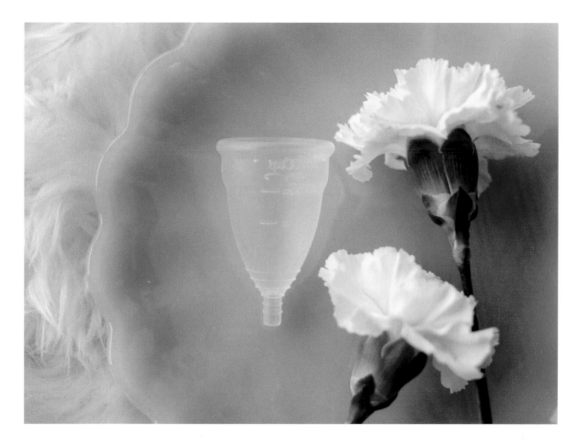

kidneys, and other organs all have to deal with them, too.

Lighten your overall toxic load by being mindful of what you allow in your personal-care and beauty routines. The Environmental Working Group's website, ewg.org, is a great place to start if you want to research this topic or particular ingredients further.

PERIOD CARE

Healthier period products have improved by leaps and bounds in the past decade. What you use for menstrual care is a personal choice.

If you choose to use tampons, buy organic if possible. The cotton in tampons is (obviously) inserted into one of the most sensitive parts of your body where there's a highly absorbable membrane. Chemicals, pesticides, and bleach used in conventional cotton can be absorbed into the bloodstream.

An alternative that works for some women is a silicone period cup. Personally, I was hesitant to try this, but now I'm so glad that I've made the switch and feel it works better for me. Aside from much less waste, one of the biggest advantages is that it can be left in for up to 12 hours. Just like a tampon, a period cup may still present the possibility of toxic

More Simple Ways to Healthify Your Home Environment

- Keep a few live plants around. Live plants not only purify the air in your home, from an energy and feng shui perspective they literally bring your space to life. Don't have a green thumb? Try succulents. These little plants are super easy to care for—just give them a splash of water about once a week and put them in a sunny spot.

- Use an essential oil diffuser to add natural essential oils into your home's air. While not strong enough to physically detox anything, these aromatics work on a sensory level and can improve your mood. You may find peppermint or citrus energize you, while eucalyptus and lavender can be calming. Some oils are poisonous to pets, so take caution if you have fur friends in the house.

- If you like candles, burn natural ones made from 100 percent beeswax, soy, or other natural ingredients. Avoid candles made from paraffin wax as these can release highly toxic benzene and toluene into the air, both known carcinogens.

- Open your windows or doors even just a crack to allow fresh air to breeze through your home. Toxic fumes that you can't detect are released over a period of years from paints, finishes, and varnishes, and fungal spores and dust mites circulate through almost every space. The air we breathe indoors is often more polluted than that of the outside, even if no odors are present.

- If possible, use a vacuum with a HEPA filter or an air purifier to remove allergens, dust mites, and other microscopic particles that can cause allergic reactions or skin sensitivities.

shock syndrome, so read the package insert and use it as directed.

Newer versions of period panties—panties designed with built-in absorbable padding—are also an option. It's estimated that if a woman selects tampons or disposable pads that she'll use—and dispose of—more than 10,000 in a lifetime. Just like plastics, these end up in our landfills and oceans. Silicone cups and period panties are reusable options, and I'm sure inventive people will come up with even more alternatives in the future.

Again, menstrual care is a personal choice. Stay mindful and pick the healthiest and best option for you.

Chapter Summary

- Your health is more than what you eat.

- Healthy habits build on each other.

- Your physical environment influences your food choices because environmental cues trigger certain behaviors.

- Healthy kitchen tools are made from nonreactive materials such as wood, bamboo, stainless steel, cast iron, or food-grade silicone.

- Detoxing harmful chemicals from your cleaning, laundry care, and beauty products can help to lessen your overall toxic burden.

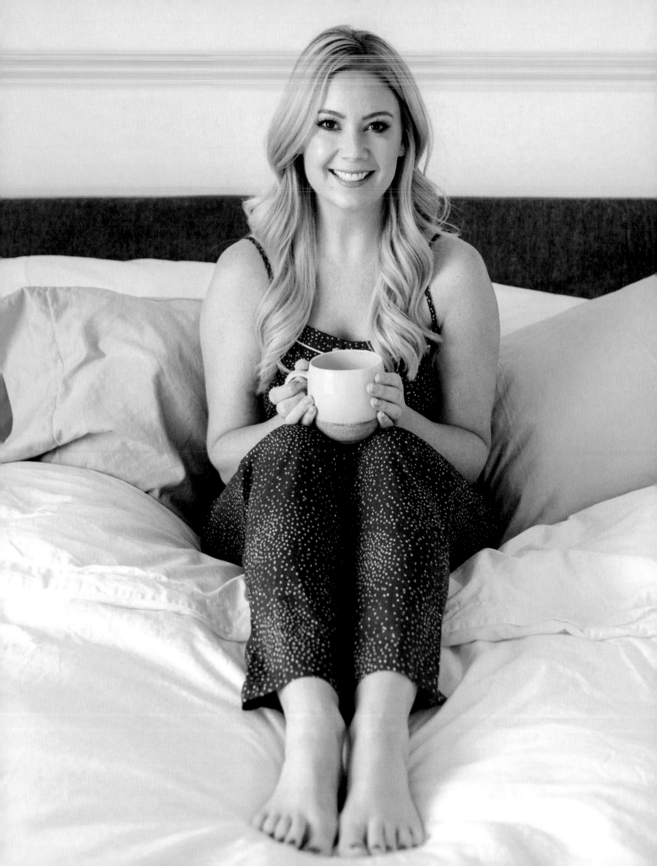

CHAPTER 6

The Bookend Method

You cannot pour from an empty cup.

Self-care. *Mind-body connection. Wholeness.* All of these words are thrown around a lot in the health world. But sometimes the real message gets lost because, as the person craving better health, you might be misled to believe there is a right or wrong way of doing these things.

Self-care doesn't have to be a luxury spa date or $30 exercise class. If trying to keep up appearances and posting validating images of all of your self-care stresses you out, then it's working against you, not for you.

Self-care is anything that nourishes your soul and helps you become an even better version of yourself. You can also consider things like talking to a life coach, going to a therapist, or having a good long cry over the phone with a friend as self-care.

Self-care is an agreement with yourself to take time to replenish. It's taking care of your wholeness, body, mind, and spirit. Getting a pedicure with toxic lotions and polish while listening to gossip TV filling your brain with other people's problems may not be the best thing to nurture your whole self. On the other hand, taking a walk in nature, without any media in your ears, might give you the silence and space you need to hear yourself think.

A few years ago I was sitting with some friends on the last day of a business trip. One of the guys piped up and said, "Liz, this whole self-care thing that women keep talking about is completely selfish. They need to give more and be of service to people. That's where the real purpose in life comes from."

I paused for a moment and said, "Chris, what did you do this morning?" He replied, "Woke up, went for a run, then wrote my daily goals and got to work." I had my answer: "Yes! You engaged in a healthy amount of self-care so you could take on your day and be of service to other people. Meanwhile, your wife woke up and immediately made the kids breakfast, then checked her e-mail to see if anyone in her circle of friends and family needed anything. She stuffed the classroom goodie bags, wrote out the grocery list, piled the kids into the car,

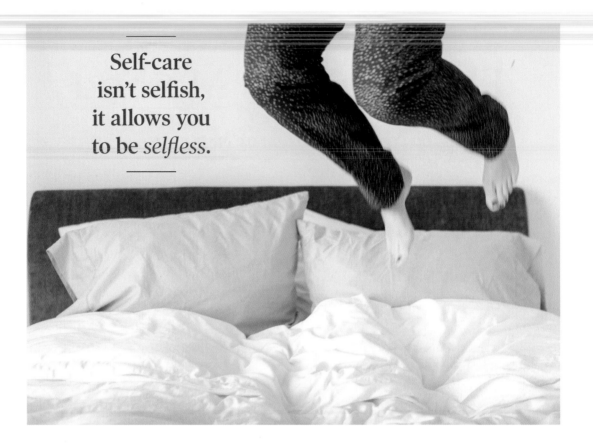

Self-care
isn't selfish,
it allows you
to be *selfless*.

and her day took off. By 2 P.M. she probably hadn't even brushed her hair."

After a minute, Chris said, "But that's just how she is." Then we had a real conversation, with the rest of the group joining in. How women tend to take care of everyone else before prioritizing themselves because they feel like they have to. How women feel like they need "permission" to do things for themselves.

I know that this is a gross generalization, and I'll leave further dissection of men versus women for another book. But I've found it true that most women are wired to take care of everyone and everything around them before taking care of themselves, while men seem to

know innately that they need to take care of themselves so that they can take care of other people.

This is where we women need to have the discipline to take care of ourselves so that we can take *better* care not only of our own minds and bodies, but of everyone else around us, too. You cannot give what you don't have.

The discipline of your Health Habit isn't about not eating a certain food, it's about taking time to set yourself up to want to take better care of yourself. This is where self-care comes in. If you're checking e-mails, catching up on work projects, planning Pinterest-worthy meals, cleaning the house, or doing

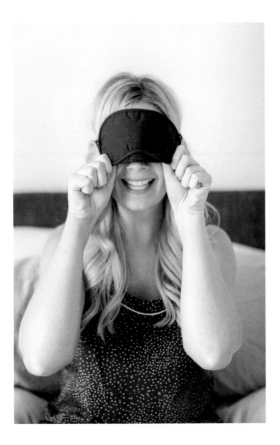

Your daily habits occur in cycles, which turn into both physical and emotional habits. When you don't slow down to connect with yourself and feel an inner sense of peace, these cycles can become long bouts of eating away your feelings or sabotaging all of your good efforts with food or drugs that you know do not serve you. Self-care increases your self-awareness, and self-awareness is the first step to feeling free in all areas of your life. Remember when we talked about freedom way back in Chapter 1? Freedom comes from the self-awareness of the beliefs, habits, and circumstances that are holding you back.

When you have self-awareness, you have the key to begin to make positive change. As you engage in deeper levels of self-care and gain more self-awareness, you'll become more aware of what's triggering your feelings.

Remember, you are not your feelings. Feelings occur in a moment in time—but if you aren't willing to pause and identify why you feel a certain way, it can become an automatic next step to use food to reverse a negative feeling. If you can identify why you feel bad (e.g., overwhelm, contempt, frustration, sadness), then you can consciously shift away from eating your feelings.

For instance, if you want to eat the entire pantry shortly after you've had dinner, it's easy to both overconsume and berate yourself for doing so. Instead, if you can, get into the habit of pausing to check in with yourself and ask, *Where is this stress coming from? What happened at work yesterday that is making me feel so overwhelmed?* or, *What underlying expectation do I have of my partner/child/friend that I don't feel is being met right now?*

other chores before you've taken care of you for the day, then you're guilty of this, too. Self-care isn't selfish, it allows you to be *selfless*.

Self-care is an agreement with yourself. It's a commitment to take time to fill your mind and body with nourishing foods, thoughts, and deeds. Self-care can be as simple as a hot Epsom salt bath, reading a fantastic book, having a long chat to connect with a friend, or taking the time to prep some yummy (and healthy) food for dinner or the rest of the week.

Taking care of yourself sets you up to make better choices throughout the day, and it's your daily routines that create your Health Habit.

Negative feelings and emotions aren't bad—they are warning signals that you need to make a shift. This isn't about being positive in a fake way, it's about being mindful and learning to use food to fuel your cells and body instead of as a temporary distraction from negative feelings.

But, you may well ask, *how do you do that?* It's way easier said than done, right? The first step is to refocus your daily habits on self-care, rather than your endless to-do list.

When you fill up your cup first, you can pour into others, and have enough left over to pour into yourself. You cannot pour from an empty cup. Eating your feelings away stems from running on empty. It's like trying to shake that last drop of water—or, who am I kidding, coffee or wine—from the cup and feeling bummed that there's nothing left. At that point, you know you have to fill it back up if you want more.

Yet, when it comes to what we can give, we constantly empty our cups but expect them to never run out. Just as important as defining your eating style, it's absolutely critical to your well-being to consciously craft self-care practices that work for you. If your self-care goes by the wayside, your health goes by the wayside, too. And—trust me—that never-ending to-do checklist filled with showing up at social events, shopping for another wire basket for your pantry, or perfecting your kid's Halloween costume isn't as important as you think it is. None of that stuff really matters if you don't feel well.

It all starts with taking control of your day, so your day doesn't control you.

If you don't have your health, everything feels hard. When you have your health, you can accomplish anything. This is how sustainable health works; when you finally surrender to self-care you'll have more than enough to pour. Your cup will overfloweth and you'll be strong enough to share yourself with others, too.

THE BOOKEND METHOD

The most tangible way I've found to help women—and myself—engage in nourishing self-care is through a flexible and individual practice that I call The Bookend Method.

Bookending your day with self-care simply means that you have a morning ritual and evening ritual that fills up your body, mind, and spirit. It's giving structure to your Health Habit by establishing non-negotiables tailored to creating the physical and mental environments for your health to flourish. When you start and end your day with these kinds of rituals, not just your health, but your *life* will flourish.

If you just rolled your eyes at me and thought, *Who has time for this crap?* then, honey, I suspect you're one of the ones who needs it the most. Instead of resisting, try digging deep and believe that you are worth taking care of.

That's the question: Do you feel worthy of taking better care of yourself? And yes, that's a really big question. If I were asked that question in my 20s, my answer would have been, "Of course!" In my 30s, it's more, "Um, I think so, but I'm not sure, but I think I can get back to that." And if you've ignored that question for decades, you probably have a big stone in your throat right now. Because if you haven't thought about it for a long time, the answer might be "I'm not sure" or even "No." And that's okay.

No matter where you're at, you can get back to feeling worthy of filling up your cup so you can pour into others. Stick with me, and stick with this book. Together, we are going to make it happen, because if there is anything I know for sure, it's that you deserve vibrant health.

Remember how we spoke about setting goals to achieve desired results? Once you identify vibrant health as your desired outcome, you can set the goals to make that happen. And once you make these actions into a ritual, you're on your way to establishing your Health Habit.

It all starts with taking control of your day, so your day doesn't control you. A morning self-care ritual will look different for everyone. I'm going to give you some great ideas, but only you know what will fill up your proverbial cup.

For example, my friend Jen is a success entrepreneur who journals and meditates for 90 minutes every single morning before doing anything else (yes, people like this exist!). When I told my working-mom-with-two-kids sister about Jen, she was like, "WTF, who has time for that?!"

For my sister, a morning self-care ritual is waking up 30 minutes before her children, committing to no phone time before 8 A.M., and doing 15 minutes of online workout videos followed by 5 minutes of breathing exercises to center herself before her day takes off. If she can do that five days a week, her days are calmer, more focused, and (no surprise here) she puts better food in her body.

Both morning rituals serve different women with different lives. The point is to create time and space for self-care at the beginning of your day, because how you start anything sets the tone for its outcome.

This is why you'll see theater casts, football teams, and yoga classes have prayer and intention circles right before the big show (or game or class). It's why people go to church on Sundays—be it an actual church, family Sunday Fun Day, or other form of devotion—and why Meal-Prep Sundays are so effective. It's why we set resolutions and goals in January. And it's why a morning ritual is critical to actually enjoying your healthy habits.

How you start your day influences how you will make decisions until the next cycle begins. And when you start by filling up your cup, the rest of your healthy habits will become actions you look forward to, not something you dread.

Your Morning Routine

I think the perfect formula for a stellar morning self-care routine starts with the physical basics, such as tongue scraping, natural skincare, and hydration; moves on to a mental practice like journaling, meditation, or centering breathing; then adds something physical such as walking, stretching, or yoga; and ends with nourishing low-glycemic food and any supplements you take to start your day off right.

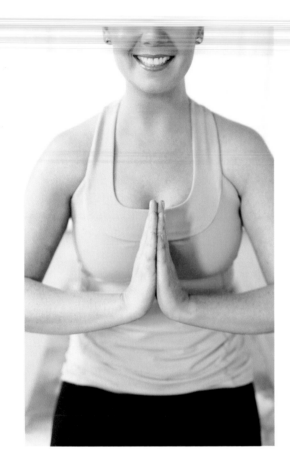

This, of course, is just a suggestion. There is no wrong way to do it, as long as your routine serves your highest good. I do have a warning, however: Don't force every single self-care routine known to woman into your mornings and evenings, because obsessing about doing it all or, worse still, doing it all "right" will stress you out and defeat the point.

Also, it's healthy to mix things up! If you've only been praying or meditating, try some journaling to uncover thoughts that want to be written. If you only stretch in the morning, try adding in a brisk walk to get your heart pumping and blood circulating.

If you don't have a routine yet, start with the rituals that are the most appealing to you, and give them a chance to become habits. You don't need to be rigid, you just need to be consistent about taking care of yourself.

Remember, consistency beats perfection every time. Feel free to see what works best and let your morning and evening rituals adapt with the seasons of the year and the seasons of your life.

What follows are some more examples of morning self-care rituals. Pick the ones that feel right for you:

Meditation is scientifically proven to improve your health. A general goal of meditation is not to have a blank mind, it's to observe your thoughts without judgment. You don't need any special equipment, just some time and quiet(ish) space.

Sit up in a comfortable position, usually on a cushion to allow your hips to be a little more open, and take long inhales and exhales as you clear the chatter from your mind and listen to what your body and spirit want to tell you. Start with 3 minutes, then increase to 5, 10, and up to 30 as needed and feasible.

Prayer is a personal preference. Prayer taps you into what you want in life and allows you to receive intuitive guidance. Even if you're not religious, you can still pray. Your desire for something better for yourself, someone else, or the world is a prayer.

It's impossible to pray incorrectly. You can pray to God, pray to your highest self, pray to our Universal Connection, pray to Mama Earth, or pray to the thought of something bigger than yourself. Prayer has been around

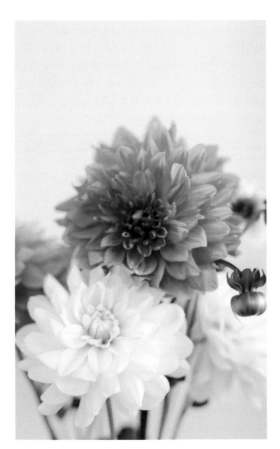

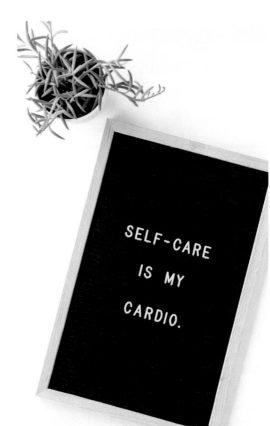

since the dawn of time and was not invented by any particular religion (despite some of them making you feel that way).

No one has the corner on or claim to prayer. It's your birthright and you can do it in any way that suits you.

Journaling is hands-down the simplest way to fast-track your growth. Plus, along with prayer and meditation, it's free. Just like you can't pour from an empty cup, you can't allow more in your head without getting what's already in there onto paper.

Journaling can be a form of self-therapy and allows your brain to uncover thoughts and feelings that don't come out verbally. I suggest handwriting your journal as much as possible because the tactile connection of your mind to hand to paper allows for free-flowing thoughts. Let your journaling be stream-of-consciousness style. You can write in bullet points, paragraphs, notes, or sentences. Don't overthink it, just get all of your thoughts onto paper no matter how messy it might seem. The more you do this, the easier it gets. I've included some journaling prompts in the 28-day kick-start at the end of this book to get you started.

Practicing gratitude can show up in meditation, journaling, and prayer, but I want to specifically call it out here.

Until two years ago, I didn't get why people needed a gratitude ritual. I'm a grateful person by nature. I love people like crazy, let them know it, and don't take the positive experiences in my life for granted. I already felt super grateful, so why did I need a ritual? It felt like another thing clamoring for space on my already-too-long to-do list.

Taking time to write out what I'm grateful for felt kind of pointless. But I was wrong. Dead wrong. I went through a low period when I felt something was lacking. I knew it had nothing to do with material goods, but the feeling was still there. I didn't have enough time, and I had too many demands. My endless to-do list added to this feeling of lack no matter how many things I checked off. Then I carved out a little gratitude ritual, and it brought immediate relief! Like taking your bra off at the end of the day relief—it felt that good.

A gratitude ritual immediately shifts you from what you *don't* have to what you *do* have. And when you feel stressed, a shift is exactly what you need.

A gratitude practice can be as simple as taking two minutes to handwrite 10 things you're grateful for. Anything that comes to mind is fair game. The "big stuff" like health, spouse, family members, and the "small stuff" like almond milk lattes, the awesome new playlist for your workouts, that you could afford your dentist appointment this month, or the fresh air while you walk your dogs.

The most important thing in your gratitude ritual is to be as specific as you can. Instead of "I'm grateful for my sister," try "I'm grateful my sister called me on my way to work and really listened while I told her about my disastrous date last night."

Take it up a notch by focusing on feelings rather than events. Like, "It felt great to banter with my sister about dating in the modern world." Write as many as you can in the allotted time (you may well find you want to keep going, and that's okay too!). If you're ever in a hot mess of a spot mentally, do this exercise for immediate relief.

Breathe. Yes, this is something you do already, but you can turn it into a mini self-care practice. Similar to a meditation, a breath practice calms your nervous system and increases oxygen in your body. Increased oxygen not only boosts your energy, but it also boosts your body's ability to detox.

Begin by sitting comfortably while paying attention to each inhale and each exhale. Start with 2 minutes and increase to 5 or 10 as needed.

Read a positive or uplifting book for 5 to 15 minutes. *The Alchemist* by Paulo Coelho, *You Can Heal Your Life* by Louise Hay, *Option B* by Sheryl Sandberg, *The Big Leap* by Gay Hendricks, *The Four Agreements* by Don Miguel Ruiz, and *The 5 AM Club* by Robin Sharma are some of my favorites.

Gentle yoga or deep stretching not only keeps you mobile so your body can keep up with life, it doubles as a form of meditation or prayer. That is, after all, what yoga essentially is: a combination of physical poses (called asanas),

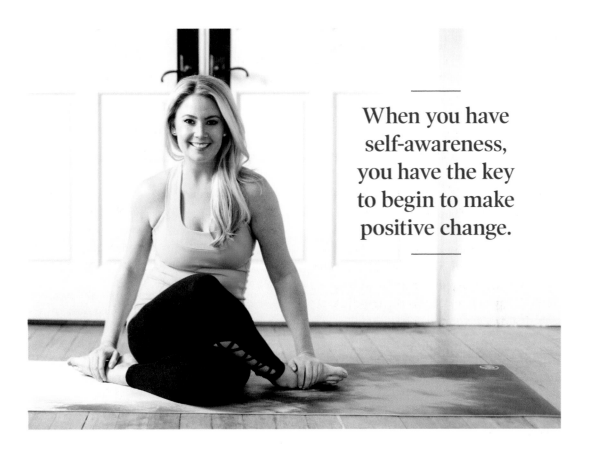

When you have self-awareness, you have the key to begin to make positive change.

with breathing techniques, moral disciplines, and mindfulness of self (in total, called the eight limbs of yoga).

Rehydrate your body with 20 ounces of filtered water. Your body functions miraculously on its own, pumping your heart, breathing, and maintaining 37 billion chemical reactions per second to keep things humming along. (Isn't it amazing that we are even alive?) The one basic necessity it can't do for itself is rehydrate.

Every cell in your body needs water to function, so keep up with your water intake so it can do its thing. (See page 65 for more information.)

Eat wholesome, natural, low-glycemic foods, which at breakfast time usually includes eggs, naturally raised meats, whole-rolled or steel-cut oats, high-quality protein powders, whole fruits (not fruit juices), low-sugar fermented foods, nuts, seeds, and vegetables or no-sugar-added green vegetable juice.

As a quick reminder, the most common high-glycemic food culprits include anything made with flour or processed grains; fruit juices; coffee creamers containing any amount of sugar; most other things with added sugars; and anything with artificial sweeteners. Ditching these high-glycemic foods in the morning is absolutely critical to your health.

Here are the things that stay constant in my morning routine—I've been doing them for so long that I'm on autopilot:

- I list three things I'm grateful for, right when I wake up.

- I take my thyroid medicine and chug 20 ounces of filtered water before anything else to rehydrate from lost moisture while sleeping (chugging is a personal preference; sipping is probably better).

- I apply nontoxic face moisturizer to rehydrate from the night before (I shower and wash my face after exercise, but still moisturize right when I wake up because it feels good).

- I brush my teeth with nontoxic toothpaste and use the tongue scraper before I do anything else (because, hey, when you work from home your self-worth goes in the toilet if you're in your jammies with yucky breath all day).

- I change my clothes, usually from sleeping jammies into yoga pants (aka professional jammies).

- I make my bed, which is a proven habit to kick-start a chain of other good decisions throughout the day.

- In recent years, I've become dedicated to no screen time during the first hour of my day, as well as 10 minutes of yoga-style stretching, deep breathing, and journaling or reading in the morning. I mix those things up

depending on how I'm feeling. In some seasons I commit to journaling 30 days straight, in others I read for 10 minutes to start my day with a happy heart.

- Four to six days per week, I do 30-50 minutes of some type of vigorous exercise, such as running, walking, weight circuits, or hiking.

- Finally, I break my fast with a low-glycemic breakfast no matter what. It's either eggs or black beans with an almond flour tortilla and hot sauce, or a healthy smoothie with one serving of pea protein, half of a frozen banana, about one-third cup of other fruit, and a teaspoon of hemp or chia seeds (see the recipe section for ideas). I take my vitamins and supplements with my breakfast, before I start my day.

Apart from the exercise, all of this takes about 30 minutes to an hour, and sometimes less. I even do it while I'm traveling. I'm not perfect, so even if I can do three or four of those things I know I'll have a good day.

You might already do a lot of these things in the morning and just need some tweaks to make it into a consistent routine with mindful choices, such as using nontoxic products and adding some mindful stretching or journaling to ground yourself. You might be able to squeeze your routine into 20 minutes, and you might include way more than I do. None of that matters.

What matters is that you consciously set yourself up for a good day. If you wake up,

Consider a Spirit Corner

Last year as I was unpacking in my new space, I started setting meaningful items on a little wood table in the corner of my office so they didn't get lost or donated. When I was done, I realized I had a special little corner of my most sacred items. A crystal my middle sister gave me from her trip to Sedona, a "little sister" book from my eldest sister, a brass singing bowl that I found in a tiny shop in Bali, another crystal from my business mentor, a few other meaningful trinkets, and my very first Bible that my grandmother gave me when I was seven years old (pink, with my handwritten "my frist [sic] bible." Turns out spellcheck is my saving grace as an author.).

I decided to leave it all there and dedicate that area as a sacred space where I can sit and center myself. I added a small cushion and find myself sitting there often to journal, pray, or to simply breathe in peace and collect my thoughts.

I don't consider myself a particularly religious person; because my heart feels that every belief system has it mostly right, I don't subscribe to just one of them. Just like my eating habits, my spirituality doesn't need to fit in a labeled box. Dubbed my Spirit Corner, this has been one of the most joyful parts of my living space ever since.

check Instagram the second your eyes open (hello, comparisons), down a blueberry muffin chased by orange juice (whoa, high blood sugar), then start e-mailing or working before taking time for yourself, mindfulness goes out the door and you're going to be frazzled, reach for the quickest food possible (hey, fast-food drive-through!), and feel like you don't have enough time to get anything accomplished. However, if you cultivate your morning in a way that both serves your psyche and nourishes your cells, you'll more naturally stay more focused, act mindfully, and gravitate to those yummy veggie bowls, big entrée salads, and wholesome meals that you know are better for you.

Remember, how you start your day sets the tone for all the day's choices. Commit to health in the morning and your mindfulness will blossom as your inner critic fades.

Your Evening Routine

The second part of The Bookend Method is your evening routine. Benefits of a solid evening routine include better health, slowing the aging process, less anxiety, easier weight management, and a greater sense of inner peace.

While your morning routine sets you up to take control over your day so you make better choices as you go out into the world, your evening routine grounds your physical and mental energy and winds you down to do one of

Tuning In, Not Out

In general, try to avoid screen time in your morning and evening rituals. Not only do we spend enough time on our devices, but the blue light jolts us awake. Trust me, I get sucked into cat videos on Facebook (why are they so cute?!) and a good Netflix binge myself—I'm in Season 3 of *The Good Wife* and I'm hooked—but just because a little mindless binge watching is fun doesn't mean it fills up your cup.

We all have our ways of numbing a little, perhaps having glass of wine, zoning out on a crime drama, going down the Facebook rabbit hole, getting sucked into YouTube videos, or even eating something on the naughty list (treat yo' self!).

I think it's unreasonable as a health coach, and a citizen of the planet, to expect that you or I won't ever do any of those things ever again. It's human to want to check out a little bit. But it becomes troublesome when your go-to numbing mechanism becomes your only source of pleasure and self-care.

If you need to numb big time every day—be it with six fast-food tacos, an entire bottle of wine, or a dozen double-chocolate brownies—it's no longer just a little deviation from your Health Habit, it's an unhealthy reliance on numbing away your thoughts to ignore what's really going on. As we've already discussed, when it comes to food, "eating your feelings" is generally a result of letting your self-care and mindfulness go.

A healthy self-care routine doesn't tune you out, it tunes you *in*.

the most critical things your body needs to get and stay healthy: sleep. And not just any sleep, but a restful night's sleep. Before we dive into a doable evening self-care routine, let's talk about the glorious benefits that only sleep can give you. Sleep is the best drug on the planet. Seven hours of restful sleep every single night is the minimum your body needs to thrive.

Getting enough sleep is not a luxury, it's a necessity. It's also free and something you can't buy—although it's worth a lot. Not getting enough sleep increases your risk for chronic diseases such as type 2 diabetes, heart disease, obesity, and depression.[1]

Even though your consciousness is in slumber while you sleep, your body is actually quite active. Sleep is how the body restores itself; think of it as all hands on deck for maintenance. Your skin is repairing—or not, if it doesn't have the right nutrients—your brain is recharging, and your blood sugar is stabilizing. Without a good night's sleep to give you energy the next day, you'll have a hard time sticking to all of those healthy habits that you've been setting up so diligently.

If getting a good night's sleep eludes you, you're not alone. An overwhelming number of people—myself included—have trouble sleeping. Just like your morning routine sets the tone for your day, your evening routine sets the tone for your sleep.

Sound Sleeping Tips That Work

Stick to a consistent sleep schedule. Get up at the same time each day, even on weekends and during vacations. This tip was the hardest for me in the beginning, but had the most impact on improving my sleep. It is one of the single best things you can do if you're having a hard time sleeping.

Start your nighttime routine early enough to be in bed to get at least seven hours of sleep, and get up at the same time every morning. A little wiggle room is totally fine—you're not a robot—but your body loves consistency and routine. I used to struggle to get up in the mornings, but I now get up between 6:00 and 6:30 a.m. daily and without an alarm.

Remember, consistency beats perfection, so if you sleep in a little one day, don't fret, just get right back on schedule.

Establish an evening self-care routine in an environment that relaxes you and preps you for bed. Use your bed only for sleep and sex (unless your go-to sex spot is somewhere else, then just use your bed for sleep).

Work, phones, computers, or other devices do not belong in the bed and using them there creates a habit loop that works against good sleep. And yes, television is included as one of those devices. Sorry to those of you who love

to fall asleep to your TV, but your mitochondria (the energy centers in every cell in your body) can even detect blue light through your skin! I know that sounds a little sci-fi, but it's true. Even if your eyes are closed or covered and you can't "see" the light, your body still knows it's there and it disrupts your restful night's sleep.

Remember, you get to choose if you control your devices or if they control you. I know, that sounds hard. But it's not as hard as struggling through your day because you sabotaged your good night's sleep.

Keep the room at a cool, comfortable temperature. You'll sleep more soundly in a cool room because your body temperature naturally drops while you sleep. If you've ever tried to sleep on a blistering summer night without air conditioning then you know what I'm talking about.

A cool room between 60 and 70°F initiates better rest. Use blankets to stay comfortable—you shouldn't feel freezing—but your body will more naturally adjust to the right temperature in a cool room. Depending on where you live this may or may not be difficult; just do your best. I set the thermostat to 64°F in the cold months (it might snow sideways overnight and I don't want it too low), and use air conditioning or fans in hot months.

Limit exposure to bright light in the evenings, especially the blue light emitted from your computer, phones, TVs, and other screened devices. Blue light is scientifically proven to

> # Sleep is the best drug on the planet.

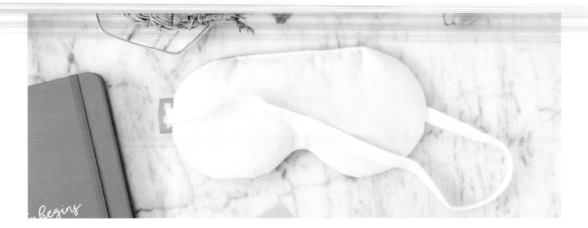

keep you up at night, but you may not notice it as it doesn't even look blue.

Blue light looks like other light and is everywhere; it even comes from the sun. Light-emitting diodes (LEDs), used in energy-efficient bulbs and devices such as smartphone screens, also contain blue light. I promised to not overload you with science so I'll just give you one quick fact: Blue light has a short wavelength and produces more energy than lights with longer wavelengths, like red lights. The problem is that LEDs and devices are mostly just blue light, and don't contain the red, infrared, and violet light that the sun also emits.

Your brain can't handle such an overload of blue light without the others, hence, the excess blue light is called "junk light." Even your skin can sense blue light with your eyes closed like I mentioned before, which is why it's crucial to sleep in a dark room; no TV, no streetlights shining in, and no digital clock or other random lights if possible.

I realize that not everyone can sleep in a pitch-black room; just do the best you can to eliminate or reduce any light in the room while you sleep. I put black electrical tape over the light on my fan and use an old-school analog alarm clock with no light if I need an alarm.

Eat dinner at least two hours before bed, and eat enough to fill you up. Active digestion right before you head to bed diverts your body's energy to digestion instead of repair while you sleep, and takes away from your body's natural healing process.

Eat enough at dinner so you don't feel hungry before bed, and load up on good fats at dinnertime, as they satiate you and give your body slow-burning fuel. Salmon, eggs, grass-fed beef, bone broth, avocados, healthy oils, nuts, and seeds all contain good fats.

If you are hungry after dinner, eat a light, healthy, no-added-sugar snack such as nuts or a small low-glycemic meal. Popcorn, juice, toast, cookies, or muffins will only raise your blood sugar and prevent restorative sleep. Air-popped popcorn on a Friday night while you watch a family movie or people-watch downtown with friends? Not a problem after a wholesome dinner. Popcorn every night for dinner? You'll have blood sugar issues that'll keep you up and sabotage your health.

Try a nighttime elixir of raw honey with apple cider vinegar. An hour before bedtime, mix one tablespoon of raw honey with one to two tablespoons of apple cider vinegar in about one cup of hot (but not boiling) water.

Honey has been used for centuries as a sleep aid. Choose raw honey as it will have more enzymes and be less processed. Hot water will kill some of the enzymes in both the honey and apple cider vinegar, but it doesn't ruin all of their nutritional benefits (this is why we use hot, not boiling, water). I boil water in my electric kettle and let it sit for 5 to 10 minutes before using it.

There aren't any scientific studies as to why this nighttime drink works, but it does. Some nutrition experts hypothesize that raw honey replenishes liver glycogen more efficiently than anything else, which allows you to stay asleep longer. Try it and see if it works for you. (See page 173 for recipe.)

In addition to the things listed above, exercising regularly, maintaining a healthy diet, avoiding caffeine after noon, and reducing your fluid intake right before bed (as that might cause you to wake up in the middle of the night to use the bathroom) will also help you maintain good sleep.

Along with a whole host of natural health benefits like more stable blood sugar, improved cognitive function, and increased longevity, sleep is also your most powerful natural beauty tool. Two weeks straight of a no-added-sugar eating plan and a good night's sleep every night and your friends will think you got Botox, or extra Botox if you already get Botox.

Here is an example of an evening self-care routine that will set you up for success.

STARTER SELF-CARE EVENING ROUTINE

2 TO 3 HOURS BEFORE BEDTIME	Finish a healthy dinner rich in good fats. Sip on herbal tea—I like peppermint or lemon balm—before bed if you crave a treat.
1 HOUR BEFORE BEDTIME	Turn off all screens and LEDs lights and dim all other lights. Turn your thermostat to a cool temperature if needed.
55 MINUTES BEFORE BEDTIME	Prepare a hot Epsom salt bath with 2 cups of Epsom salts and a few drops of your favorite essential oil (I prefer lavender); the magnesium in the Epsom salts will help relax your system, and soaking in the hot water will help ground your energy; or read to your kids or connect with your partner. Or, do whatever fills up your self-care cup and calms your mind. If desired, take a melatonin or magnesium citrate supplement to aid your sleep even more.

Melatonin is a naturally occurring hormone in your body that regulates your circadian rhythm; it's also an antioxidant. As a supplement, it can help make you sleepy and fall asleep more quickly. This over-the-counter supplement is generally considered safe and non-habit forming when taken in small doses. Start with 0.5 milligrams and take up to 2 milligrams if needed according to the package instructions. I think melatonin is best used occasionally, but work with your health-care provider if you have questions.

Magnesium is a vital nutrient that every cell in your body needs to thrive. It also works as a light muscle relaxer and can aid in the feeling of relaxation by counteracting feelings of stress to give you a more restful night's sleep. I especially appreciate how it calms my jittery leg muscles at night. But because it's a muscle relaxer, it can cause a little too much relaxation in your colon, which can lead to many trips to the bathroom.

Just like melatonin, start with a low dose and add more as needed. Magnesium citrate is easy to find in powdered form at the natural foods store and easily mixes with water. There are other forms of magnesium, such as magnesium glycinate, that also work well. Try them out and see what works best for you. They are generally safe for everyone, but if you're taking any prescription medicine be sure to check with your health-care professional before adding this or any other supplement to your diet. Even "natural" drugs are still drugs, and can interact poorly with other medication.

But what about sleep aids, you might ask? Well, short-term sleep aids—either over-the-counter or prescription—for emergency situations, like an acute injury or a once-in-a-decade awful sinus infection—are most likely not going to harm you if recommended by a health-care professional. But relying on over-the-counter or prescription sleep aids over the long haul is detrimental to your health.

Especially beware of taking antihistamines, such as Benadryl or NyQuil, for sleep. Antihistamines are indicated for short-term use for things like itching, severe allergic reactions, and allergies. While they might make you drowsy, the sleep quality is usually not great and, more important, they are habit-forming and come with serious side effects in the long term. Moreover, most over-the-counter sleep aids are antihistaminic drugs repackaged and labeled as something to help you achieve sleep, but they're not any better.[2]

Just like everything else you have to swallow, your liver and other detoxification organs have to process these sleep aids, which can cause additional stress on the body. In lieu of pharmaceutical sleep aids, try a dialed-in evening self-care routine that contains a mindfulness meditation or potentially melatonin and the tips I mentioned above.

Kava and valerian root are two additional natural herbal sleep remedies you can try if needed, but they should be taken in the short term, as the safety of long-term use of them on the liver has not been established.

Your morning routine sets the tone for your healthy day, and your evening routine winds you down and preps you for sleep. Both can take just a few minutes or as long as 90 minutes—only you know what works best for your schedule. The most important thing to do here is mindfully incorporate both into your day.

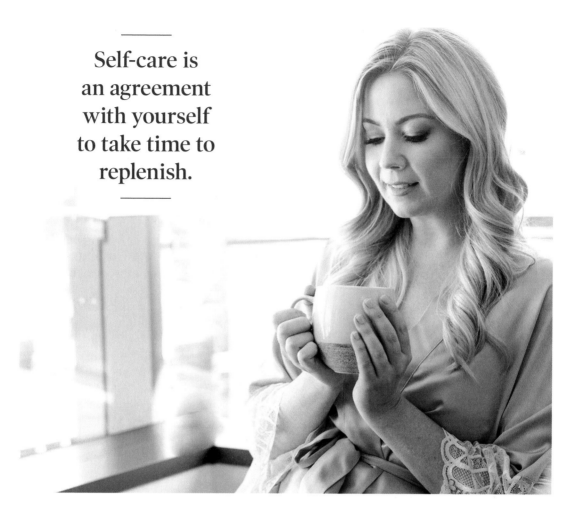

Self-care is
an agreement
with yourself
to take time to
replenish.

These new bookends will do wonders for your healthy habits, thus your overall health. When you start the day mindfully taking care of your health, you're going to look forward to continuing to nourish your body. That spring greens salad is going to look way better on the menu than the highly processed preservative-laden bread. A cup of hot tea will sound way better than office-grade coffee with powdered creamer (what is in that stuff, anyway?!).

But the self-care doesn't have to stop there. Once you get your bookends established, you'll be ready for more. Self-care doesn't have to be a broken record of doing the same thing over and over again, or a $15 Tibetan-yak-tear-infused bath bomb. As I mentioned before, it can be anything that tunes you in to becoming the healthiest, most content version of yourself.

Allow your self-care to shift and grow during the seasons of the year and the seasons of your life. Here are a few ideas to get you started:

- Prepare yourself a nourishing homemade meal.

- Take a yoga or meditation class.

- Go for a long nature walk.

- Wash your face and apply nontoxic skincare lotion.

- Take a hot salt bath surrounded by dim light or candles.

- Have a spa treatment.

- Dry-brush your entire body, starting at the feet and working toward the heart.

- Journal about what you want your future to look like.

- Drink no-sugar-added green juice.

- Dig in the dirt.

- Read a soul-nourishing book.

- Take your vitamins and supplements.

- Use a foam roller to roll out your facia.

- Oil pull (rinse your mouth with coconut oil for 20 minutes).

- Meditate.

- Declutter and donate or gift things that no longer serve you.

- Book your annual physical (making the appointment counts!).

- Visit a local hot springs.

- Apply a natural face mask and have a long phone chat with an old friend.

- Learn about *hygge* (the Danish word for intentional coziness at home).

- Handwrite 100 things you're grateful for.

- Watch an uplifting movie.

- Enjoy a raw vegan dessert.

- Create a "Stop-Doing" list (Buh-bye endless to-do's).

- Take a solo mini vacation or staycation.

- Go to a play or live theater performance.

- Spend an hour doing your most beloved hobby (garden, play piano, etc.).

- Take a nature hike.

- Take yourself out to a nice meal.

- Go for a long bike ride.

- Write a list of intentions or affirmations.

- Have a cozy lunch with your BFF or spouse.

- Give up alcohol for the weekend.

- Attend a church or spiritual service.

- Take a tango or other dance lesson.

- Have sex! Sexual intimacy and pleasure release feel-good hormones that can help manage cortisol levels.

- Watch the sunrise.

- Watch the sunset.

- Listen to gentle music while you stretch.

- Make your bed.

- Tidy up your space.

- Do your breast self-exam.

- Exercise with mindfulness.

- Partake in anything that fills up your proverbial cup but doesn't drain your health.

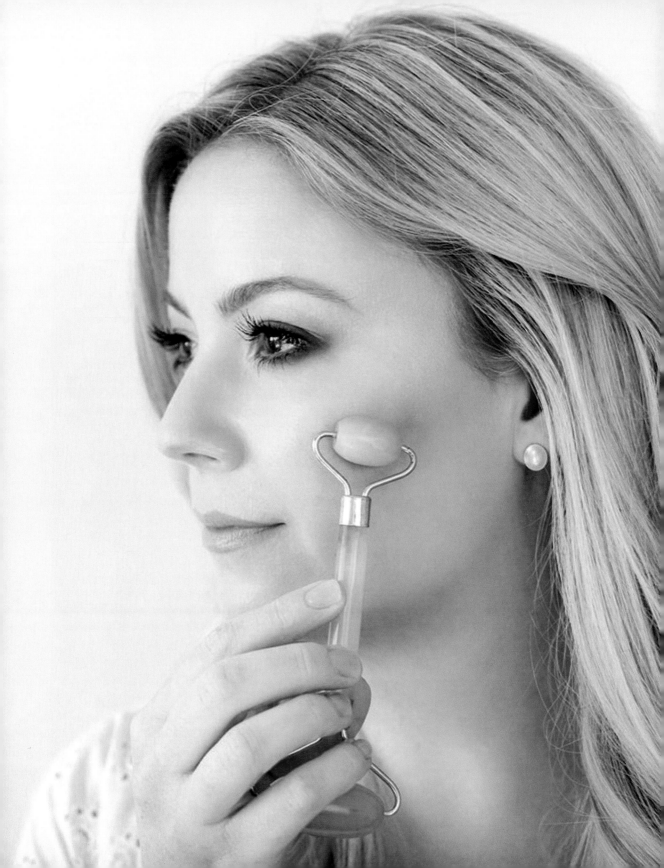

WHAT ABOUT EXERCISE?

You might be wondering where exercise fits in to all of this. After all, a gentle walk outside or light stretching is excellent for your body, but it doesn't necessarily get your heart rate up or build muscle.

I left exercise routines as the final section in this chapter because I've noticed with my clients how a consistent exercise routine often becomes more manageable after the food and self-care pieces are in place. When someone comes to me and says she can't lose weight despite "working out all the time" I'm never surprised.

Rushing around stressed all day and fitting in a stressful workout just for the sake of burning calories typically doesn't lead to weight loss, it leads to . . . more stress. Moreover, exercise is usually the thing that gets left off the list if your day is running you, or you may be too tired to even think about a workout. Exercise isn't any less important now that you know how to fill up your cup, and it is something you will look forward to when all of your other habits are in place.

You can add daily exercise into your morning routine, or fit it in where it works best in your schedule. The Mayo Clinic recommends 30 minutes of moderate physical activity every day, while the CDC and American Heart Association both recommend at least 30 minutes of moderate physical activity five days per week.

This means that at minimum, to maintain your health, you should get your heart pumping for at least a half hour most days. Remember, your goal is consistency, not perfection.

Speaking from Experience

I used to lie awake in bed as my mind would spin on every e-mail I forgot to send (did I ask my web designer to use the image with the blue shirt instead of the green shirt?), what I didn't buy at the grocery store (crap, I'm out of oats and I forgot the crackers for the party tomorrow), or feeling guilty for not calling a friend back (ugh, I hope she knows I care).

Even worse, I'd wake up the next morning and check Instagram first thing, then read e-mails on my phone before even sitting up. My day started off with cortisol through the roof and feeling the weight of the world on my shoulders. It felt like I couldn't make progress in anything. I couldn't focus, no matter how much green juice I had during the day.

After implementing a diligent evening self-care routine, I started to fall asleep with peace.

And guess what? I still had the exact same amount of e-mails when I checked in an hour later than usual. And the feeling of missing out on Instagram went away. My days are easier, and my stress levels are dramatically lower. Aside from an inexpensive melatonin supplement and some yummy nontoxic face cream, my new routines didn't cost me a dime.

My new life motto is good nights equal good mornings, and I'm sticking to it.

You can even break your half hours of moderate activity into smaller or longer sessions.

As the saying goes, the best exercise is the one you do, not the one you think about doing. So if you don't love the thought of an intense 30-minute sweat session, the goal of walking 10,000 total steps per day also has dramatic health benefits. Studies have shown that hitting 10,000 steps per day can reduce blood pressure and increased sensitivity to glucose[3] (which is a good thing and wards off diabetes).

Do what works for you, just make it a habit to move. Everyone has different body and physique goals. If you love weight training, specific sports like tennis or surfing, salsa dancing, or endurance training, then do those things. Do more of them! Just like creating meal plans, there isn't just one best way. The amount and intensity of your exercise habits will change with your age and seasons of life.

There is a wide array of what can get your heart pumping, from a brisk walk or jog uphill, to swimming and surfing, to power yoga, to dance or Jazzercise (had to throw this in for the baby boomers). Studies show that 30 minutes of moderate exercise each day yields dramatic health benefits. Take note of the word *moderate*; you don't have to kill yourself in a boot camp or run a marathon to reap the benefits of exercise.

It's not an all-or-nothing kind of situation. Ten minutes of mild exercise strengthens connections and communication between memory-focused parts of the brain in healthy young adults.[4] This means even a short period of mild exertion can yield considerable cognitive benefits, and the results showed immediately afterward.

Additionally, a study published in the *American Journal of Hypertension* found that 61 to 90 minutes of exercise a week was more effective at lowering systolic blood pressure than just 30 to 60 minutes a week.[5]

If you need ideas to get your heart pumping, look outside. Nature gives us incredible natural terrain in every corner of the world. Have an ocean or a lake? Go swimming (safely). Live by a hill or mountain? Take a walk uphill. Flat and snowy? Cross-country ski. Flat and warm? Go for a jog. Join a gym or find an exercise class that excites you.

Personally, I like the combination of two weight-training workouts, two high-intensity interval sessions (HIIT), and one yoga class per week. That schedule keeps my energy high and body lean. The two benefits you want to see from exercise are that it raises your heart rate and builds or maintains muscle. Raising your heart rate comes from moving fast, such as steady-state cardio, HIIT, or plyometric moves. Building or maintaining muscle comes from resistance training, either from your body weight through pushups and the like, bands used to create resistance, or lifting weights. Circuit training involves moving fast through exercises and uses weights or body-weight resistance that can double as cardio and strength training.

If you're a yogi and the style of yoga you practice keeps your heart rate up and maintains muscle, then that's a perfect choice for you. If you prefer hikes out in nature, your heart will pump in the fresh air and moving uphill will build muscle. If your walk involves mainly long flat stretches, perhaps add some lunges, squats, and pushups for some resistance.

Benefits of Exercise:

- Improves insulin sensitivity, reducing your risk for type 2 diabetes

- Releases endorphins—the feel-good neurotransmitters—and boosts your mood

- Helps balance all of your hormones, including the stress hormone cortisol, which we all need help managing

- Increases circulation for glowing skin and more mental clarity

- Removes toxins via sweat and increased circulation

- Can boost your metabolic rate, which can help you maintain more lean body mass

- Lowers your risk of breast, colon, and endometrial cancers[6]

If you're curious about how much you need to exercise to lose weight, remember that exercise is about 10 to 20 percent of the weight-loss equation. The rest is food.

You can't exercise away poor eating habits. If you've been spending hours in the gym but haven't seen a change, the answer is changing the way you eat (and balancing your hormones through stress-reduction and potentially supplements), not exercising more.

Which leads me to some helpful guidelines about how to fuel yourself for exercise. If you're simply walking or doing light exercise to get your heart rate up, just eat as normal. If you're doing some type of intense athletic training, work with an expert in your field, as there may be specific sports-nutrition requirements.

If you're performing an intense workout that includes weight training, HIIT, or endurance sports, the guidelines for eating around exercise don't change a lot from general healthy guidelines discussed in the previous chapters. Eat a small meal that contains a good carb, a high-quality protein, and a small amount of good fat within 30 minutes of finishing your workout. You can also have a similar meal or snack before your workout if that feels best to you, however a meta-analysis of 46 studies suggests that your body burns more fat if you work out in a fasted state, provided that your workout is less than 60 minutes.[7] If you're endurance training for more than 60 minutes, a small pre-exercise meal or snack can enhance performance. In the same study, pre-exercise eating had no effect on HIIT.

Working out in a fasted state generally means that you exercise in the morning, before you've eaten anything. This works for some people, but if you feel light-headed, are too hungry, or exercising for more than 60 minutes, then eat before you work out. Regardless, save the majority of your healthy fats for the opposite time of day as your workout, not close to your workouts.

Fats are slow-burning and best kept for the meals that are not near your workout during the day. That doesn't mean to skip the fat—every meal and snack should have a little—it just means to not overload on them right before or right after a workout.

The carbs are a better fuel source for your workout. For example, two scrambled egg whites with one whole egg and veggies, some overnight oats with a small handful of nuts, or a protein smoothie with half a banana and a half teaspoon of flaxseed oil are all great pre- and post-workout meals. A whole avocado, salmon, or grass-fed beef or other meals higher in fat are best left for another time of day not close to your workout if you want to dial-in on fat loss and exercise performance.

Now, you know how important exercise is, but how do you actually make it happen consistently? For me, I always think about the phrase, "I regret the hour I just spent exercising, said no one ever." In all seriousness, the discipline of exercise doesn't necessarily come from actually doing the workout, it comes from being willing to put on your exercise shoes and get out the door. That's always the hardest part.

If you've been in a phase without exercising, first, be gentle on yourself. Then commit to getting your shoes on and getting out the door. Take those first steps—you won't regret it.

Chapter Summary

- Self-care is an agreement with yourself to replenish your mental, physical, and emotional energy, which allows you to show up more in every area of life.

- The Bookend Method will help you craft morning and evening rituals that will help your healthy habits. A morning self-care routine sets the tone to make healthy decisions for the rest of your day.

- An evening self-care routine helps wind down your energy and ground you to prepare for a good night's sleep.

- Exercise benefits all areas of your health and should include things you enjoy.

- When you fill up your proverbial cup first, you can pour into others, and have enough left over to pour into yourself. You cannot pour from an empty cup.

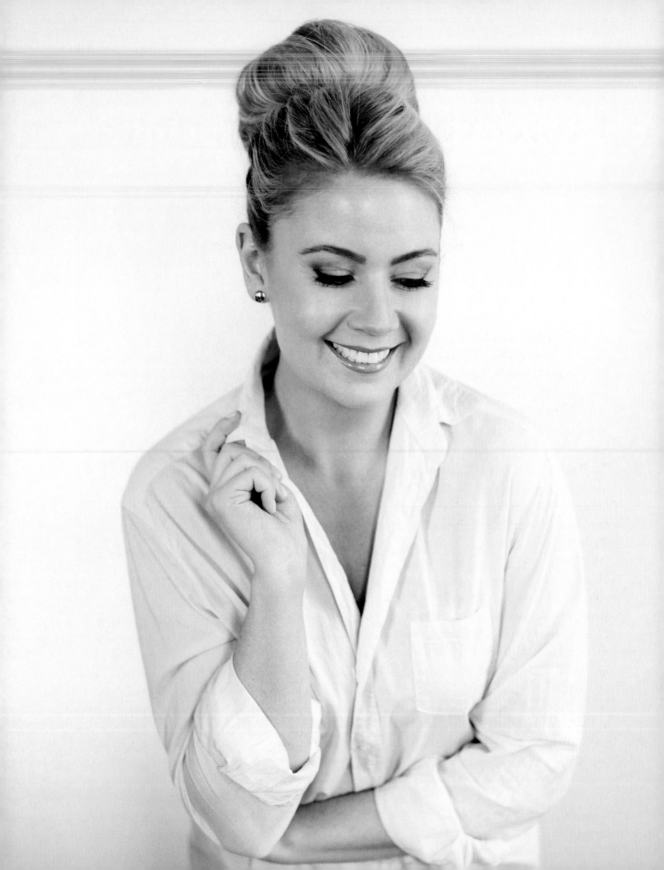

CHAPTER 7

Uncover the Intangibles

Don't let these sneaky tricksters
defeat your healthy habits.

I f I had a dollar for the number of clients who have said, "Just tell me what to do and I'll do it," then I'd have enough money to have fresh green juice delivered to my house every day for the rest of my life, with enough to spare for all the bath salts and lavender drops I go through faster than toilet paper.

Women have a tremendous amount of will, and ultimately we can stick to anything for a period of time. Show up for a gut-wrenching exercise class five days a week with the intention of rocking a bathing suit over spring break? Yes, we can! Follow an elimination diet to a T and eat celery while watching our family and friends gorge on creamy artichoke dip with perfectly toasted crusty bread right in front of us? Yep! We will not break. Starve ourselves while diligently following a tough intermittent fasting schedule? Most can will it into existence.

So why, if we can do these things as we're told and not cheat, do so many of us still not reach our health goals? Or worse, slide

backward? I've got news for you: It's not that you don't want it badly enough (I know you do) or that you're not strong enough (I know you are) or that you're doing it wrong (you're not). It's that there is something intangible affecting your health goals, and it ain't gonna uncover itself on its own.

This is the part of creating healthy habits that people like to skip. It's like hiking up a 14,000-foot mountain and taking the trolley for the last 500 feet because that steep, jagged terrain at the top looks tough and you might get hurt. But if you do that, you'll miss out on the best part of the journey, the one that teaches you the most.

For many, uncovering the intangibles is the hardest part of the process, because even seeing the connection between what we're about to talk about and your health is a leap of faith. But don't fret, I'm going walk you through it so it feels easy peasy. Okay, I kind of lied here because I want you to keep reading.

Truthfully, this might be hard; but trust me, don't skip ahead. This step might just

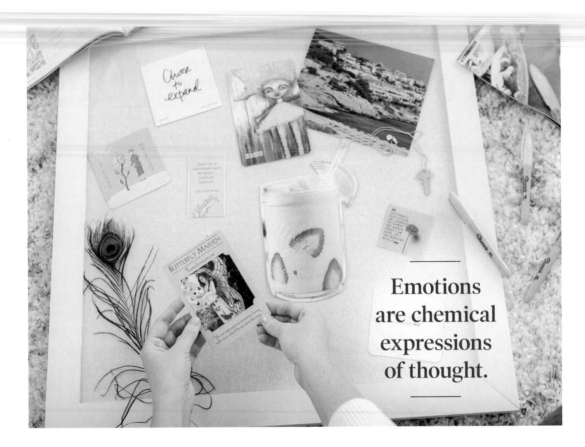

Emotions are chemical expressions of thought.

create the breakthrough you need to finally meet your goals and kick your bad habits to the curb. However, it's way less hard than ignoring this stuff forever and not achieving your goals. That part is truer than true.

It's time to meet the intangibles. The intangibles are the nonphysical, not-so-evident aspects of your life that affect your health and trigger healthy—and unhealthy—habits. They're similar to everyone's favorite superhero family, the Incredibles, in that they are powerful and can come out of nowhere, although they don't wear cool costumes and you don't always look forward to seeing them.

The intangibles affect our health just as much as the food we eat. You can have the best of intentions and a "diet plan" all set up, but the stress from non-food sources can knock the wind right out of you and force a bag of Cheetos and a dozen cupcakes down your throat.

Remember way back in Chapter 1 when we talked about the habit loop? As a refresher, the habit loop consists of the *cue* (aka trigger), the *action* (aka routine), and the *reward*. The intangibles are often buried in understanding the reward of why we partake in certain habits. If you still find yourself eating that pint of ice cream every night, seek to understand what type of emotional, or intangible, reward that behavior is delivering. Perhaps it's pleasure or comfort. Perhaps it's your way of checking out for 20 minutes to avoid frustration.

Uncovering the intangible cues and rewards you experience may be the final piece of the puzzle that you've been looking for. While each of these non-food sources deserve their own books—and there are thousands on each—here I'll simply set you in the right direction, then let you continue to work with them in the best way for you.

There are four intangible areas of life that I notice affect my clients' health the most (in no particular order):

1. contentment in relationships

2. happiness in career or purpose

3. positive self-talk

4. openness in belief systems

When these things work in harmony, our health flows in harmony. But when awareness around these things has been brushed under the rug for years, our health suffers.

Emotions are chemical expressions of thought. We experience emotions as physical sensations. The feeling of a tickling stomach on a first date. The knife in our hearts when we go through a breakup. The holy-cow-I'm-gonna-throw-up sensation before walking onstage.

When we experience any emotion, it starts with a thought. Thoughts spark a chemical reaction in our brains, then we feel the emotion. Once that physical process is in place, it can affect any system or cell in your body.

For instance, you have the thought of seeing your new husband for the first time after being away for a week on a business trip. That thought sparks a chemical reaction in your brain that you perceive as joy, or maybe even sexual excitement. Feel-good neurotransmitters such as serotonin are released and along with the feeling of joy, your cortisol level is lowered and your body benefits from the fresh release of the happy thoughts.

On the flip side, the thought of getting through another day of a job you hate sends the stress hormone cortisol through the roof, affecting not only your ability to sleep well, but your motivation to exercise, eat right, and so on. It also causes your brain to look for food as pleasure, which might be the reason you have an overwhelming need for a pint of mint chocolate chip ice cream every night.

Even a happy relationship or successful career can cause these unhealthy stress levels. Your physical body can't distinguish between the stress of running from a tiger versus the stress of signing your first book deal and then realizing you've agreed to work for someone else for the first time in 10 years when you cash their check, then further realizing they like to use words like *deadlines* and *due dates* (hi, Hay House!).

That's right, stress is stress to your body, no matter where it comes from. I've met countless über-successful entrepreneurs who can't seem to stop binge eating; and how many brides are stressed out of their minds on what's supposed to be one of the happiest days of their lives?

Negativity doesn't just come from bad situations. As we learned in Chapter 6, negative thoughts—and their subsequent emotions expressed as chemical patterns—show up when your cup is empty, not necessarily because the circumstance is bad.

In no particular order, these are the most common intangible areas in which my clients and program participants have had major breakthroughs:

Contentment in Relationships

Relationships come in all shapes and sizes, and include your significant other if you have one, family, friends, social acquaintances, workmates, and others. For our purposes, let's concentrate on the relationships that affect your health goals.

Think about the five people you're closest to or spend the most time with. Do healthy habits flow when you're around them? Do you feel supported in your choices? If the answers to those questions are no, that's okay. You don't have to ditch your close personal relationships, but finding new social groups with like-minded people can go a long way to feeling more content and connected.

Expressing your truth and desire to feel more supported in your healthy habits to those closest to you is another step you can take to improve this area of your life.

Happiness in Career or Purpose

Don't mistake *career* and *purpose* for believing you have to have society's version of a dream job to be healthy. Your purpose generally comes from how you spend your days; it doesn't matter if you're a CEO or stay-at-home parent.

Feeling that your time is being well spent goes a long way to creating an environment to allow your Health Habits to thrive.

And then there's the most important relationship you'll ever have you in your life. Nope, it's not your current or future spouse or children. It's your relationship with yourself and your ability to recognize negative self-talk, stop it, and reframe it.

It's pretty hard to make good decisions and stick to your Health Habits when someone is constantly saying mean things to you (and that mean person might be you!).

Openness in Belief Systems

Belief systems encompass everything from spiritual and religious beliefs to what we believe is possible for our lives and the world around us. When you're unwilling to change your belief systems and make a change if needed, you're living in fear. When you're willing to let your beliefs evolve based on new life experiences, you're living in love.

Living in fear keeps your body in a constant state of stress, which lets unhealthy habits thrive. Living in love frees your emotions and lets you accept life as it is, which allows healthy habits to form.

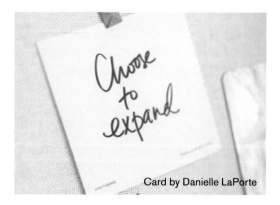

Card by Danielle LaPorte

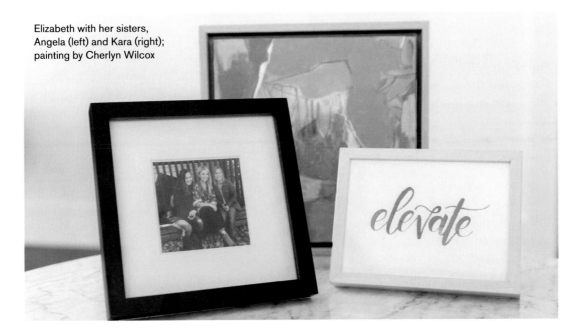

Elizabeth with her sisters,
Angela (left) and Kara (right);
painting by Cherlyn Wilcox

For each of these areas, do a check-in by completing the exercises I give you for your journal (see page 126), and revisit them often. Just like muscles don't stay fit if you don't work them, these areas of your life don't work for you if you don't give them attention.

The biggest mistake people make when starting on a personal discovery path is that they think they only have to do the work once. That if they break through a fear or work through an issue, it's fixed forever.

The truth is that, just as we can't just change our eating or exercise for one day a year and expect it to become a habit, we can't evaluate this stuff once and then never think about it again. But the more you give these areas attention, the easier it gets.

And just as with the tangible things such as goals, food, and numbers, the aim with the intangibles is consistency, not perfection; you don't have to strive for perfection in every area of your life. (Remember, perfection doesn't exist—at least not in the long term.)

Awareness is what you're looking for. Self-awareness will help you decide to do what's next. Progress over perfection wins with the intangibles.

If you want to meet your health goals, check in with each of these areas and look for ways to make progress toward feeling more content and at peace in each. The best way I can help you is to give you journal prompts so you can check in and discover the intangibles on your own.

You're the only one who lives in your head, so you have to be the one to do the work to uncover them. Journaling more, engaging in mindfulness practices, and the guidance of a licensed therapist, health coach, or life coach can also be beneficial in this process.

Speaking from Experience

Up until a few years ago my inner dialogue about how I ate and how I took care of my health was downright MEAN. I knew what to do—how to eat right, exercise, breathe, and focus on personal growth—but it was all so external.

I was so nice to everyone around me, but I never looked at how nasty my inner dialogue was, even when I was doing things right. I would berate myself for not being perfect, eating perfect, looking perfect, and anything else my inner brat could find wrong with me.

It wasn't until a few years ago that I finally started to focus on being kinder to myself instead of being what I thought as "perfect." Then something amazing happened. Everything changed.

Before, no matter how well I did things, I never had that overall sense that everything would be okay, that everything IS okay. But when I started putting more effort into being kinder to myself, that huge weight of negative self-talk and inner meanness was lifted, and it was way heavier than any external stress.

Being kind to yourself is a daily practice—it's so easy to slip into old habits—but it's genuinely the most important step I've ever taken to feeling content on a daily basis.

Boundaries:
MY FAVORITE WORD, EVER

Before we get to the journaling exercise, I want to give you a useful tool to implement in these areas that will help you improve any area of life. Meet my friend and most favorite word of all time: *boundaries*.

I discovered the concept of healthy boundaries while I was going through divorce. It was the single most effective concept that kept me sane and helped me move forward. Healthy boundaries seem simple at first glance, but they expand far beyond learning to say no and not being nosy.

Healthy boundaries are a two-way street, but you don't need the other person's buy-in to make them work. It's the awareness not to allow people to cross your boundaries, and not to encroach on other people's boundaries yourself.

For example, if you're in the middle of a breakup, healthy boundaries help keep other people's opinions or external gossip from swaying you into a decision you know isn't right for you. On the flip side, if one of your close family members or friends is going through an upheaval, telling them what they "need to" or "should" do may be overstepping boundaries (if they didn't ask point-blank, and even then, proceed with caution).

Developing healthy boundaries can be more of an art than a science. It doesn't mean that you don't care or offer support, and it doesn't mean that you should alienate people. Having healthy boundaries means knowing how to draw a firm line between what emotions, thoughts, and feelings are yours, and what emotions, thoughts, and feelings are theirs.

A few years ago I hosted a health retreat in Mexico with a group of 14 women from around the world. This was the first time I'd met any of them in person, and naturally it took everyone a while to warm up to each other. We spent the first three days and nights learning about physical health, like digestion, detoxing, and meal planning.

I always open the last and final night to the intangibles. One woman who I'll call Tracy mentioned, "Well, I hadn't thought about it until now, but maybe my eczema is coming from stress, not from diet?" Now, Tracy is one of those people most women aspire to be. She follows a no-sugar, clean-eating lifestyle diligently, exercises regularly, and reads every health book under the sun. She pulled up her sleeve so I could see it: horrible eczema. "I follow every eczema diet protocol to a T and use all of the natural remedies, but it keeps getting worse. I've literally tried it all."

I asked, "So what's going on at home?" She took a long pause, then replied, "My daughter is getting divorced and we threw her a $25,000 wedding less than a year ago. She is making the biggest mistake of her life! If I could just help her see that she is doing the wrong thing, our family would be back to normal. She came from parents who have been married 25 years, we have no idea where this came from. We are so embarrassed."

"That sounds stressful," I said, then followed with "What's your relationship like with your spouse right now?" "We hardly talk," she said. "He goes to the TV room every night and

> ## Self-awareness will help you decide to do what's next.

I shut the door because the news is so biased and depressing, so I just do my own thing." "When did the eczema start getting worse like this?" I asked.

It finally dawned on her. "About six months ago when this all began." Now, it's not that Tracy shouldn't show concern for her daughter, or that this situation doesn't sound great for anyone involved. It's that Tracy was so

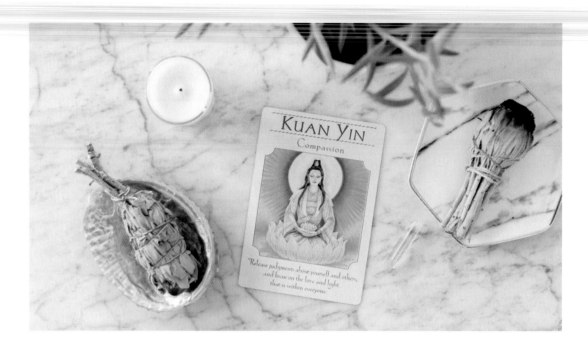

wrapped up in her daughter's decisions—which ultimately she has no control over—she was making herself sick. Not to mention possibly ruining her relationship with her daughter, and allowing friction with her own husband. Tracy hadn't drawn a boundary between what was hers and what was her daughter's. I suspect the flip side was also true if her daughter wasn't able to draw a healthy boundary with her mom.

Look, we can only set intentions and work toward what we want. Life can be messy and beautiful at the same time. The script we write for it rarely works out as planned, but that doesn't mean it's not good. In fact, once the trauma of change is past, what happens next might be even better, for all involved.

Learning to identify what you can control, and letting what you cannot control be, is often the first, biggest step toward freeing up some space in your mind to create healthier habits. Trust that change—even unexpected change—will work out in your favor.

If you need some direction for healthier boundaries, helpful words to say in a situation like this include, "What can I do?"; "I'm here to listen without judgment"; or "I care about you and I'm concerned that perhaps you have not thought about this consequence" (then genuinely listening without judgment). These are examples of support with healthy boundaries.

Examples of unhealthy statements include, "You should not get divorced"; "You suck and are making the worst decision of your life if you follow your instincts"; or, "God won't love you if you do that." These happen when you are without boundaries and project your own emotions onto someone else.

You can't control how other people treat your boundaries, but you *can* control your own boundaries and what you do or do not let in.

Establishing healthy boundaries will set you that much closer to meeting your Health Habit and achieving vibrant health for good. It also frees up space to make better decisions throughout your day.

Carrying other people's issues around weighs you down more than a hundred pints of chocolate brownie ice cream ever will.

When you begin to establish boundaries, you will start to realize how much of other people's stuff you've been carrying. I don't mean stuff like when your significant other carries your lip gloss because your dress doesn't have pockets and a jacket ruins the outfit. I'm referring to your judgments and views of other people's life choices and decisions (or the judgments and views that other people have imposed on you).

Letting go of other people's "stuff" is the difference between being the woman in the airport with 18 suitcases—including one just for her hair dryer that she cannot live without à la Princess Vespa in *Spaceballs*—who is frazzled by trying to load them onto a cart, or being the sleek business traveler walking effortlessly through security with just one rolling carry-on, slip-off shoes, and a pass for the fast lane. One of these women is making life way more difficult than she needs to by carrying stuff she thinks she needs but ultimately doesn't serve her, and the other has made the decision to dump the excess stuff and glide through life.

Likewise, distinguishing what's yours versus what's someone else's baggage is something

----

Worry sabotages your healthy habits.

----

you can do on your own as you grow, or seek a life coach or licensed therapist to help you identify these things. True, therapy used to be a taboo topic, but I'm going to go out on a limb here and hope that by now we all know that a neutral third-party expert (e.g., a licensed therapist or skilled life coach) is useful to anyone.

Your friends and family can also give you a useful perspective, but their views are always skewed by personal feelings, and you need to make sure they're not imposing beliefs on you that ultimately do not serve you. Gaining perspective from a neutral third-party expert is one of the most valuable things I've ever done to feel content in life, and I hope you consider it, too.

While detoxing your home environment helps you create a physical container to allow your Health Habits to thrive, clear boundaries create a mental container that puts you in a position to make decisions that put your health first.

THE STATE THAT ALWAYS SABOTAGES

Making healthy choices is always done in the present moment. If you're constantly living in the past or future, making healthy choices is unnecessarily hard. There's a saying that "worry is a prayer for what you don't want" and I'll extend that to mean worry sabotages your healthy habits.

Intangibles Check-In Journal Prompts

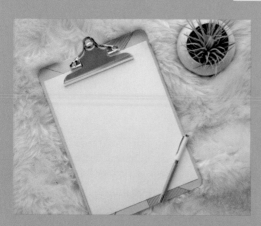

- What would you most like to do with your days?

- What resources or education do you need in order to step into a career or position (e.g., parenthood, volunteer work, job, business) that fulfills you?

POSITIVE SELF-TALK

- Are you able to observe your own thoughts without judgment?

- Are you able to recognize when your inner chatter is demeaning or mean?

- Write down any internal chatter or self-talk that you experience over the next 48 hours. What would you say to a friend if she or he were talking to themselves in that way?

- How can you show yourself more compassion?

- Write three affirmations that you know you need to hear. (If you're new to affirmations, an affirmation is a positive statement set in the present. Here are three to get you started: *I am capable of creating anything I desire. I am worthy of vibrant health. I have the tools I need for success; I lack nothing.*)

BELIEF SYSTEM CHECK-IN

- What beliefs did you learn as a child that you no longer feel to be true?

- What beliefs around success, work, and money were you taught as a child that you can now let go of?

- What spiritual beliefs do you subscribe to outwardly that you don't feel to be true in your heart?

CONTENTMENT IN RELATIONSHIPS

Think about the five people you spend the most time with.

- What are the first three words that describe each relationship?

- What patterns do you notice in these relationships?

- How would you feel differently if those patterns changed?

- How can you work toward this change?

- Where could you and the other person benefit from stronger boundaries?

- Is someone overstepping your boundaries? Or are you overreaching yours?

HAPPINESS IN CAREER OR PURPOSE

- Do you feel a sense of purpose and accomplishment in your days, that you are working toward making something that serves people?

- Does your day fuel you or drain you?

Worry comes from being in the past, which you cannot change, or the future, which hasn't happened yet. In order to shift to healthy habits, you have to drop the stories that you've already told yourself about the past and release worry about how things will turn out in the future.

Worry doesn't change the outcome of anything, it only sabotages your good intentions. If you often find yourself worrying, take a deep breath and come back to the present moment. When you live in a state of thinking about the past or present—constantly reliving a conversation with an ex, or wondering how your proposal presentation at work tomorrow will turn out—you won't have the mindfulness to make good choices in the current moment.

Does that mean you shouldn't learn from past interactions or not plan and prepare? Of course not. It simply means that good decisions are made in the present moment, and your ability to catch yourself living in the past or future and come back to the present is another useful tool in your toolbox of healthy habits. The Bookend Method and self-care practices we discussed in Chapter 6 are your best tools for staying in the present moment.

As you go through your intangibles check-ins, consider the boundaries and expectations that need to be evaluated in each. Remember, the goal of this exercise is awareness, not perfection. As Arianna Huffington says, "Life is a dance between making it happen and letting it happen." Work for progress in the intangible areas of your life, but don't forget to live.

Work on the big stuff, and don't sweat the small stuff.

Chapter Summary

- The intangibles are the nonphysical, not-so-evident aspects of your life that affect your health and trigger heathy—and unhealthy—habits.

- Your relationships, career, internal dialogue, and belief systems are all intangible factors that influence your overall health, including how you respond to stress and how you make healthy (or unhealthy) decisions.

- Aiming for perfect balance in the intangible areas of life isn't what leads to improved health. It's the self-awareness in these areas that allows you to make more conscious choices and, ultimately, more healthy decisions.

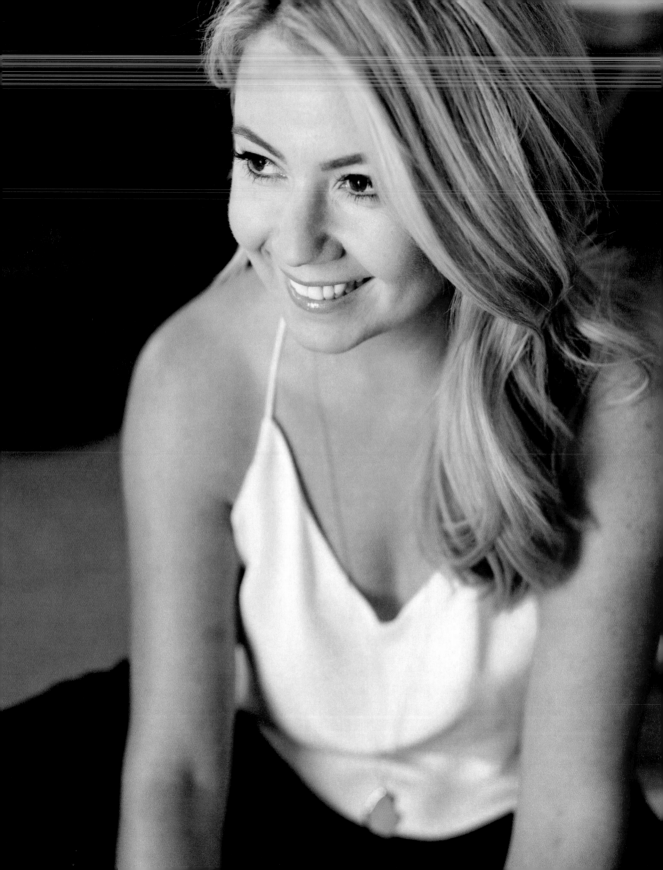

CHAPTER 8

How to Stick to Your Healthy Habits

Theory is all well and good,
but you've gotta learn how to put this into practice.

We've covered miles of ground to help you develop healthy habits that you actually look forward to. Now that you're all schooled up and well on your way to becoming the healthiest person you know, I want to give you some pretty handy tricks that you can use to stick with your new practice.

If your old habits rear their Twinkie-loving, two-pizza-eating heads, it doesn't mean that you are failing. Building a healthy lifestyle can be a two steps forward, one step back kind of process. But guess what? That's still progress, and as long as you're consistent, you can still meet your goals.

If you have a misstep, or just lack motivation on any given day, instead of feeling blue or berating yourself, remember that negative self-talk can have the same unhealthy side effects inside your body that fast food and artificially colored blue icing create.

Be gentle with yourself, take a deep breath, then get back on track. Recommit to your morning and evening routines—good health really does start and end there—and use the following tools to help stay the course.

REPLACE THE WORDS *I Can't* WITH *I Don't*

This small tweak to your internal language is scientifically proven to yield better results. Instead of saying, "I can't have ice cream for dinner," tell yourself, "I don't have ice cream for dinner." You can even add a qualifier and reframe, because hey, it's okay to have a serving of a good-quality ice cream after a healthy dinner one night each week. Something like, "I don't have ice cream for dinner, and I don't have ice cream after dinner unless it's Friday night."

Repeating "I don't" statements versus "I can't" statements can retrain your neural pathways to help you make better decisions over time.

A few "I don't" statements that help me:

I don't put any type of sweetener in my coffee.

I don't have wine on "school nights" (Sunday through Thursday).

I don't eat highly processed bread.

And trust me, I still very much enjoy myself. I love a high-quality flatbread with a glass of wine on the weekends, and I cook with things like almond flour tortillas and brown rice tortillas. There's so much good food out there to enjoy—when you crowd out unhealthy items with healthier options, you'll start to find that you like the healthier options even more.

Which leads me to . . .

USE THE *Crowding-Out Method* INSTEAD OF GOING INTO DEPRIVATION MODE

Rather than imposing strict rules on yourself, a gentle way to introduce new healthy habits is to add them in and allow them to crowd out the bad stuff. For example, instead of thinking, *I can't have any pizza on pizza night*, shift to *I always have a big, healthy green salad before pizza.*

Let the salad crowd out some of the pizza. Trust me, if you have a big, vibrant green salad (a good one—not a sad, boring one) you'll most likely be completely satisfied with one or two slices of pizza instead of six. Let a big

bowl of fresh, real food crowd out a few slices of pizza or a pot of mac and cheese.

Crowding out is often a first, best step to making healthier choices. Once you've developed the habit of crowding out, you can experiment with new types of food and ways of eating that can change your life and health forever. Let home-cooked food you love crowd out unhealthy choices.

CRAFT MORNING AND EVENING RITUALS THAT DELIGHT YOU

We covered this extensively in Chapter 6, so you're already well on your way to bookending your day with self-care that supports your healthy lifestyle. Inspirational speaker Alexander den Heijer says, "When a flower doesn't bloom, you fix the environment in which it grows, not the flower." Your morning and evening rituals create the environment that allows you to grow.

The daily actions you incorporate into your morning and evening routines can also serve as a source of pleasure (often the reward part of the habit loop), which can replace less desirable sources of pleasure like a jumbo muffin, an entire bag of chips, or a pint of rocky road with whipped topping. Pleasurable morning and evening routines will reduce the urge to use food as your only source of pleasure.

JOURNAL IF YOU FEEL STUCK

There's a saying, "The easiest thing to do is the easiest thing not to do," and it speaks to the simple yet powerful act of writing things down. Putting pen to paper solidifies your commitments by engaging a group of cells in your temporal lobe known as the reticular activating system. Your brain intensifies the amount of focus on the information you are writing down.[1]

If you ever feel stuck, get out a piece of paper and write down your health commitments. It's better to use real pen and paper instead of typing if possible as the kinesthetic movement of your thoughts adds another layer of learning to your brain. Use "I don't" instead of "I can't" statements where needed.

Even better, tape what you wrote down to your bathroom mirror, refrigerator, or vision board. Make it your phone or computer screen saver, or keep it next to your bed on a note card. Seeing your commitments and affirmations regularly creates micro visioning sessions to aid your efforts.

Which leads me to . . .

VISION BOARDS WORK

I've written about this before: Vision boards aren't woo-woo, airy-fairy exercises. Visualization is scientifically proven to work. Olympic athletes have been using visualization for decades to improve performance, and *Psychology Today* reported that the brain patterns activated when a weightlifter lifts heavy weights are also similarly activated when the lifter just imagines (visualizes) lifting weights.[2]

A vision board is one of the easiest ways to constantly remind yourself of what you want

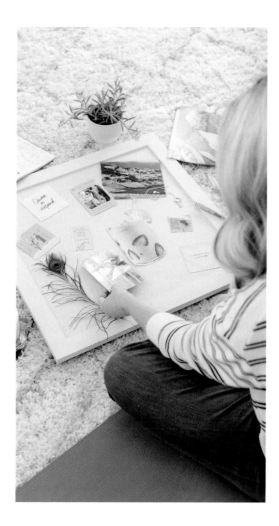

to create. In recent years, I've also adopted the idea of what I call a Spirit Corner to sit in front of as I journal and practice mindfulness and visualization exercises (see Chapter 6 for more on this).

Whether you decide to make an actual board or Spirit Corner or not, whenever you feel yourself making excuses and losing enthusiasm, take a moment to visualize what you want to achieve. Having a clear view of what you want will get you through confusing moments.

REPEAT AFTER ME: "GOOD HEALTH ISN'T ALL OR NOTHING"

If you've been doing a brilliant job of eating clean and then experience a moment of weakness, you're not back at square one. Healthy habits and willpower are just like muscles; they will get stronger and stronger the more you work them, and they will get weaker if neglected.

If you fall off the wagon, take a deep breath and hop back on without making yourself feel guilty. Neglecting the muscle once isn't what makes it weak. Neglecting it over time is the issue. Be proud of yourself for the progress you've made thus far. You're human, not a robot. Maintain your mindset of progress, not perfection.

BUILD AFFIRMATIONS INTO YOUR DAILY ROUTINE

Thinking, saying, and writing affirmations on sticky notes to be placed around your living and working space also creates mini visualizations that work. Affirmations help train your brain to make better decisions. If you're new to affirmations, check out the work of the late and beloved Louise Hay. Her book *You Can Heal Your Life* is a must-read, even if you don't think you need "healing."

Here are a few affirmations to get you started:

Healthy choices come easily to me.

I attract what I desire.

There are no roadblocks to what I want to achieve.

Good health is my nature.

I am filled with love, light, and good health.

CURATE YOUR SOCIAL MEDIA FEEDS ASAP

Follow healthy living accounts on Instagram or Facebook and subscribe to wellness-focused blogs and e-mail newsletters. However, really check in with yourself and see how you feel when you read the posts.

Last year I realized that I was following a bunch of healthy-looking accounts, but every time I saw the posts I felt like I wasn't good enough. It was a strange realization: I thought I was reading these for inspiration, but instead they were making me feel bad about myself.

Unfollow accounts that trigger feelings of unworthiness or comparison. Even if that's not the goal of the account owner (I'd say it just about never is), you have to determine how it affects you. If it doesn't leave you feeling inspired and happy, then unfollow. You are in charge of your social media feed; stay diligent on how you curate it.

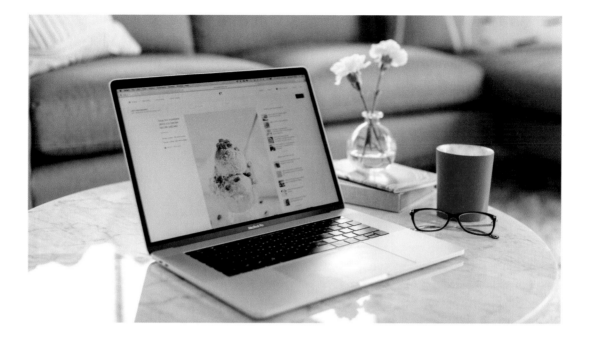

SPEND TIME WITH PEOPLE WHO SUPPORT AND INSPIRE YOUR LIFESTYLE

Make your best effort to surround yourself with people who are like-minded, supportive, and inspiring as often as possible. This might mean joining a new group in your community or online.

Take a look at the five people you are around most often and evaluate if they enable your good habits or steer you to bad choices. It doesn't mean getting rid of friends, it just means making an effort to hang with people who also get excited about lunch at a local healthy cafe or with whom you can share your latest personal growth revelation.

BE OPTIMISTICALLY REALISTIC

Goals worth achieving take effort over time. In her book *9 Things Successful People Do Differently*, Heidi Grant Halvorson writes:

> Albert Bandura, one of the founding fathers of scientific psychology, discovered decades ago that perhaps the best predictor of individuals' success is whether or not they *believe* they will succeed—something optimists do naturally. Thousands and thousands of experiments later, he has yet to be proven wrong. But there is an important and often overlooked caveat: to be successful, you need to understand the very vital difference between believing you will succeed, and believing you will succeed easily. Put another way, it's the difference between being a *realistic* optimist, and an *unrealistic* optimist.

Don't let realistic optimism deter you, though. It's a good thing and aids your self-awareness. Being a realistic optimist simply means shifting from looking for quick fixes and overnight success to appreciating and enjoying your journey, and having a realistic expectation that there will be times when it doesn't feel easy.

GRANT YOURSELF FORGIVENESS, GRACE, AND COMPASSION

And finally—and potentially most important—be gentle with yourself. It's pretty hard to make good choices when someone is constantly talking down to you.

Negative self-talk and holding grudges against yourself works *against* you, never *for* you. Same goes for forgiveness, grace, and compassion toward others. Hurtful things that have happened to you in the past are most likely not your fault, but it's your responsibility to heal them.

I call this Radical Responsibility for Self in one of the online courses I teach and it's the most popular section of the entire class. We have to take responsibility for how we handle everything that comes our way: the good, the bad, and the ugly. No one gets through life unscathed, and while many circumstances may not be in your control, how you react is. No one else lives inside your head.

Show yourself forgiveness, grace, and compassion and remember to look forward, not backward. You're not going that way.

As we wrap up, I want to leave you with this: Happiness from the inside out catalyzes actions that improve your physical health. Just like good health, happiness isn't something you achieve once, it's something you choose to work on every day of your life. Both health and happiness are more of a sliding scale than a black-and-white switch. Choose actions each day to slide both of them more toward the positive side. Be kind to yourself, be gentle with yourself, and allow for more flow and ease. Your Health Habit will follow.

Just like
good health,
happiness isn't
something you
achieve once,
it's something
you choose to
work on every
day of your life.

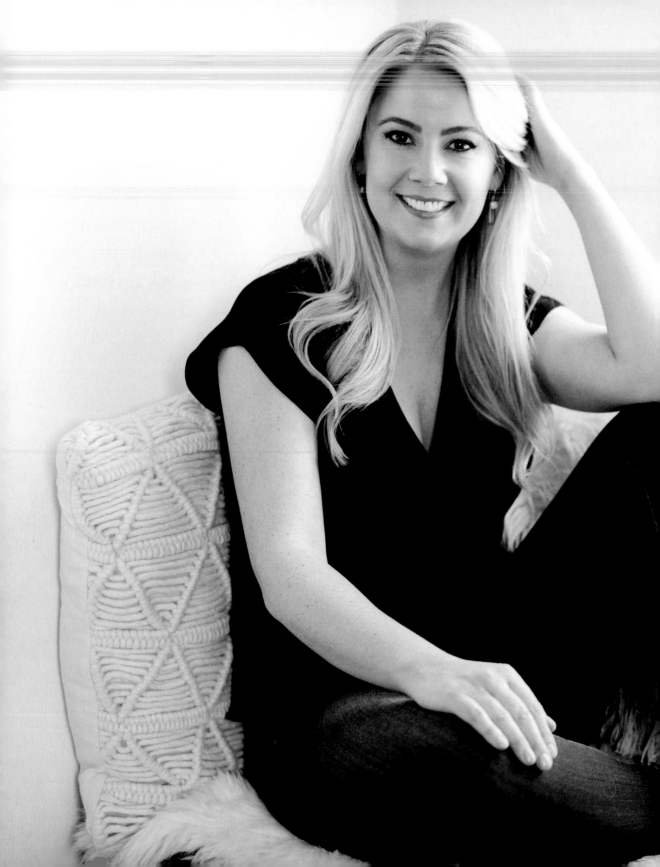

Part III

MAKING IT WORK IN REAL LIFE

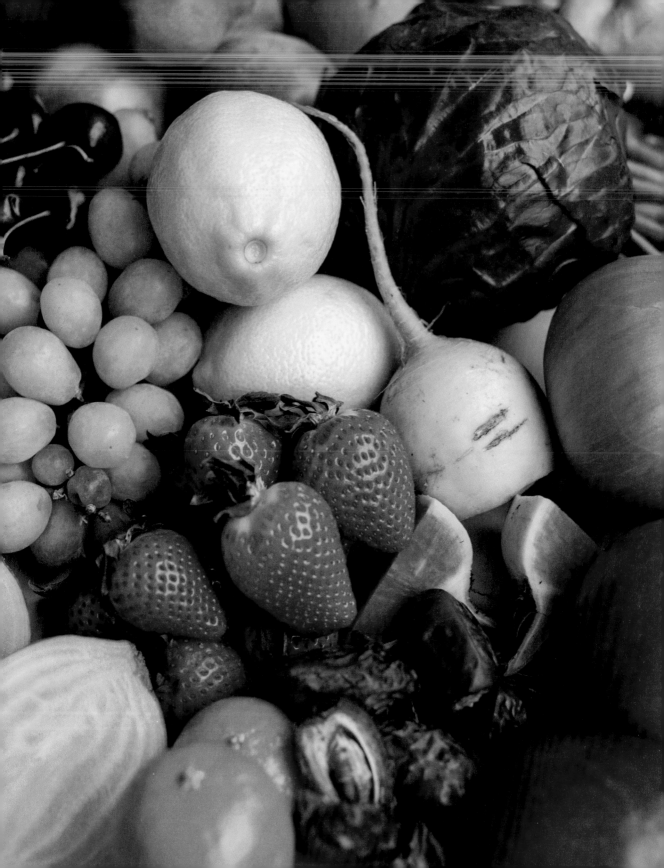

CHAPTER 9

The 28-Day Kick-Start Plan

*This flexible kick-start plan
will help you nourish to flourish.*

Psst, I've got a secret. This is one of the most enjoyable, most flexible 28-day programs you'll ever participate in. Its goal is to get you into eating delicious whole foods that you actually look forward to, while giving your body a break from the processed white flour, dairy, and excess sugar that typically weigh you down.

This is way more about what you *can* eat during the next 28 days than what you *can't* eat. It's a reset of your habits with health benefits. Once you reset your healthy habits, you'll never look back.

You can use this kick-start whether or not you want to adhere to a specific eating style (e.g., paleo, vegan, keto). If so, simply look for foods in your eating style on my "approved" and "not approved" lists and go with that. For example, if you are vegan or vegetarian, don't include the meat, fish, and/or eggs. If you're like me and you don't label your eating habits, then follow the plan as outlined; it's similar to the Mediterranean way of eating.

Regardless of what you call it, this kick-start is designed to give your body the chance to do what it's meant to do: thrive. It's all about rewiring your brain to reach for whole, nutritious foods, and to build health into your everyday life.

START WITH THE BASICS

I want to meet you where you are. I'll provide you with Level 1 and Level 2 food options, but know that Level 1 is a fantastic place to start, especially if you've ever struggled to stick to an eating plan before. Giving up highly processed gluten-containing foods and a lot of added sugars alone will do wonders for your health.

You'll also give up dairy for the 28 days so you can see if eliminating that from your eating habits benefits you or not. I'm giving you the option of eating high-quality, probiotic-rich Icelandic-style or Greek yogurt on Level 1. Your body digests these types of fermented dairy products much easier than other dairy, and they can be a good source of protein if you tolerate dairy products. I do suggest trying it without, but if you need to add it in then that's okay.

For both Level 1 and Level 2, I'm recommending you consume no more than 25 grams of added sugar each day (and you can boost your kick-start even further by consuming zero grams of added sugars for 28 days straight). Level 2 is more strict and also omits corn and soy; it's a great plan if you're curious whether these things affect you. If you've never eliminated gluten or dairy, then start at Level 1. You choose where to start, and can revisit this plan at any time. The goal of my 28-Day Kick-Start Plan is to allow these guidelines to become your new baselines. After the 28 days, if you waiver from these guidelines, you'll feel the effects almost immediately.

While at first glance a 28-day kick-start might feel restrictive, please know that there are loads of fantastic, delicious foods allowed. Don't let your mind go to deprivation. Instead, focus on all the great-tasting meals and snacks that you do get to eat: You have an abundant menu to choose from while on this kick-start.

MODIFYING YOUR KICK-START

I'm providing guidelines here, but you know you best. You can modify what you eliminate, or mix and match the meal plans and ideas to suit your needs. For instance, if you don't consume alcohol but you feel that caffeine has gotten the better of you, then eliminate that.

If Level 1 feels too restrictive, then modify it accordingly. You do need to stretch yourself a little, but I don't want you to feel too stressed or obsessive about eliminating foods from your eating plan. At the very least, eliminate highly processed grains (even the natural ones) and avoid added sugars in excess of 25 grams per day during the kick-start. If you are pregnant or nursing, or have diabetes or cancer, please check with your health-care provider before starting any new eating program, including this kick-start.

CREATING KICK-START SUCCESS

First, I'm going to assume that you've read this entire book before (or at least during) your 28-day kick-start. The information in these pages will answer just about any question that will come up.

Next, to make your kick-start as effective as possible, it's important that you prepare most of your own food, or buy it from a trusted source. Almost all packaged food is off-limits during the kick-start, as most packaged food contains excess sugars and preservatives. However, I've included an approved packaged-foods list because, hey, I'm not a monster, and I understand that you can't put your entire life on hold because kids and jobs don't stop for kick-starts.

If you do decide to buy prepared meals, become a label sleuth and read labels diligently. For example, if your local natural grocery store's prepared foods section lists the ingredients on each dish and they're in line with the guidelines, that's perfectly acceptable!

Healthy prepackaged food generally costs more, but if the ingredients line up and you can afford it, then they are okay to use. My own local market makes a black bean hummus dip and lists the ingredients as simply black beans, tahini, tamari, garlic, cumin, salt, and pepper. Spread on gluten-free almond flour crackers, it's one of my favorite snacks. However, it's pricey, so I only buy it occasionally rather than making it myself.

I've also included rotisserie chicken as an approved food for meat eaters because I know life gets busy. But if you can afford it, opt for organic, as it is usually higher quality. Remember, though, that rotisserie chickens are usually coated with not-so-healthy oils, so remove the skins.

Dining out at a chain restaurant that doesn't list every ingredient is not allowed on the kick-start—you'd be shocked at what is in this food, most of which comes from food suppliers and is just opened and microwaved in the back, like a TV dinner. Restaurants mostly use low-quality canola oil or vegetable oil—even in salad dressings—because of the large volumes they produce. It's best to skip them during your kick-start.

> ## Once you reset your healthy habits, you'll never look back.

If you can find a restaurant where the ingredients line up with the kick-start guidelines, then it's okay to use occasionally. Let your server know your dietary guidelines and don't assume that just because gluten, dairy, or added sugar isn't listed on the menu that it's not in the dish.

One of my favorite fresh authentic Thai restaurants makes a wonderful red curry dish. The menu lists coconut milk, spices, and veggies, but when I double checked with the server he told me that they do put some heavy cream (dairy) in the coconut milk curry dishes, as most American palates are accustomed to it. Apparently this is common practice in many Asian-style restaurants in the United States. I asked and they were happy to make mine dairy free. My point: Always ask.

In general, always buy the highest-quality food you can afford and make your absolute best effort to eat clean. It might seem like a stretch to omit gluten, dairy, added sugar, and alcohol for 28 days, but trust me, with all the incredible options you have to replace those things, you won't even miss them after the first few days. Except the wine. You'll miss the wine (or beverage of your choice). But do your liver a favor and give it a break. It's only 28 days and I know you can do it.

One-pot meals of hearty homemade soups or stews make for great kick-start meals, as does anything that you can batch-prepare. Always think, *cook once, eat two or three times*. If you get the food processor out to make a batch of Magic Sauce (see recipe, page 192), double or triple the recipe and freeze what you don't use for next week or the week after. If you prepare a chicken dinner Monday night, it will keep in the refrigerator for two days, so consider cooking up enough for Tuesday or Wednesday night as well. A big pot of lentil soup? Double it and freeze the rest for later. Generally, most foods keep for two to three days in the refrigerator, and up to four months in the freezer.

Frozen fruits and veggies make healthy eating simple and are budget-friendly. But remember to read the labels. For example, the ingredients list for frozen peas should be just peas. If anything else is added, move on to the next brand in the case. Frozen fruits and vegetables do not need preservatives or additives, but not every producer packages them this way. While fresh produce contains more enzymes and shouldn't be skipped, frozen produce is generally flash-frozen right when harvested and most of the nutrients are preserved. They still contain the same amount of fiber and are full of hydrating plant water.

Check the Environmental Working Group's Dirty Dozen and Clean 15 lists (ewg.org) and buy organic if you can based on these lists; just because they're frozen doesn't mean they weren't treated with pesticides.

Most canned food is off-limits because it's usually full of preservatives. When it comes to veggies, fresh is best, then frozen, and never store-bought canned. The only canned food exception is canned beans (black, garbanzo, etc.) and canned tomatoes.

Always rinse canned beans before using to remove excess sodium, and look for ones with reduced or no salt. If you can find beans or tomatoes in BPA-free cans, boxes, or other containers, even better. You don't have to use these items, but they're acceptable here.

Food that you or a local farmer canned and preserved at home via old-school canning methods—in glass mason jars with no preservatives—is absolutely allowed. If you know how to do that, congrats! I used to watch my grandmother do it and remember the loud *slup!* sound of that mason jar lid being sucked in successfully.

And finally, my best advice to find success with this program is to review the guidelines, then make a long list—the longest list you can—of your favorite foods that fit into this framework. For example, some people love pesto and some people loath it. If you love pesto, make it dairy free (see recipe, page 195) and serve it over chicken, fish, or your favorite rice noodles. If you dislike it, no need to eat it.

Love tacos? Try the Slow-Cooker Chicken Tacos (page 232). Find fish unappealing? You don't have to include it. Only you know your favorites.

Make a list of what you can have that you like to eat, identify meals that fit in, and then make a five-day meal plan that you can rotate through. From that five-day meal plan, go grocery shopping. I don't want to ask you to buy a bunch of food that might go bad or that you may never use, so I didn't include a shopping list. That's the part where you need to step in and do some of the work.

There are thousands of types of whole foods on the planet; use this time to try new things and discover new dishes you love.

Quote by Antoine de Saint-Exupéry

ADDING FOODS BACK IN

When I host wellness retreats, we follow a similar plan to the one outlined here. I call going home "reentry" into the real world. Your senses are on high alert after a kick-start plan like this.

If or when you decide to add back in foods you eliminated during the kick-start plan, it's critical that you only add in one thing at a time to recognize how foods affect you. If on day 29 you go out for an Italian dinner of fettuccini Alfredo and wine, not only are you going to feel horrible the next day from the sudden jump of gluten, dairy, and alcohol, but you'll have no idea which one of those things is the biggest culprit.

Add foods back in one at a time, and give yourself at least one full day in between. That means if you reintroduce cheese on Monday night, wait until Wednesday to add anything else back in. If you're feeling great, you may not want to change from this regimen.

If you do reintroduce foods, I suggest writing down how you feel 15 minutes, 1 hour, and 12 hours afterward to notice if you have any symptoms like headaches, skin troubles, or digestive upset. Stay mindful and go slow, especially with sugar or alcohol. Your tolerance has been reset and your liver is humming along great. Don't dump a bunch of trash into it.

28-DAY *Kick-Start* GUIDELINES

1. Eliminate the following allergens during your 28-day kick-start:

   Level 1: no gluten, no dairy, no added sugar,* and no alcohol; reduced or no caffeine

   Level 1 with fermented dairy option: no gluten, no dairy (except unsweetened Icelandic or Greek yogurt), no added sugar,* and no alcohol; reduced or no caffeine

   Level 2: no gluten, no dairy, no added sugar, no soy, no corn, no caffeine, and no alcohol

2. Start every morning with hydration. Choose either 20–30 ounces of filtered water or 12 ounces of hot water with a generous squeeze of lemon (or both) before anything else.

3. You must eat a protein-rich breakfast within the first hour of waking up. If you want a number to follow, protein-rich means 20 to 30 grams of protein.

4. Take a high-quality multivitamin with your breakfast. Also consider an omega-3 fish oil supplement, vitamin D, and a probiotic if they fit into your budget.

5. Get at least 30 minutes of moderate activity five days per week while on this plan. If doing more frequent or intense exercise, add meals and snacks as needed.

6. You must give yourself at least a 12-hour fasting window each day. That means 12 hours between the last thing you eat at night (except water and herbal tea) and breakfast, while still following guideline #3. Bonus if you can make it 13 to 16 hours.

7. Every meal and snack during your 28 days should be low-glycemic and contain a healthy protein, good carbohydrate, and good fat.

---

*At the very least, consume no more than 25 grams of added sugars per day if you feel too restricted on Level 1.

THE GOOD STUFF

EXAMPLES OF SOURCES OF PROTEIN	• Meat • Fish • Eggs • Black beans • Lentils • Quinoa • High-quality protein powder • Nuts are generally sources of good fats but also contain protein.	• High-quality soy products like tofu, tempeh, and edamame also contain protein if you choose to consume them. • Dairy products also contain protein, but we're eliminating them from this kick-start (unless you choose to incorporate unsweetened Icelandic or Greek yogurt).
EXAMPLES OF SOURCES OF GOOD CARBOHYDRATES	• Whole fruits • Whole veggies	• Legumes (lentils, beans, and peas) • Gluten-free whole grains
EXAMPLES OF SOURCES OF GOOD FATS	• Avocados • Salmon • Extra-virgin olive oil • Flaxseed oil • Nuts	• Seeds • Virgin coconut oil • Other cold press oils or fatty fish are also good sources of good fats.

You'll notice that some foods do double duty. For instance, black beans double as a good carb and a protein. Most foods contain some combination of proteins, fats, and carbs, and you don't have to obsess about it. Simply look at your meal or snack and make sure all three are present.

For example, an apple on its own is a healthy carb. Adding some nuts or nut butter would add some protein and healthy fat. Black beans contain a healthy carb and protein, so

adding some extra-virgin oil or avocado to your black beans would complete the meal.

A salad of greens and veggies is a good carb, topped with some lentils or chicken for protein and avocado or oil for fats makes a winner. There are literally endless combinations to satisfy your cravings. You'll find a bunch of examples here, too.

Remember back in Chapters 3 and 4 when we talked about fiber? Your fiber will naturally come from your good carbs (whole fruits, veggies, legumes, and whole grains), but double check that your meals are loaded with fiber, too, especially if you follow a low-carb eating plan.

Nuts also contain some fiber, but your best sources will come from leafy greens, other veggies, whole fruits, legumes, and whole grains.

LEVEL 1 APPROVED FOOD GUIDELINES	LEVEL 1 APPROVED BEVERAGES	LEVEL 2 APPROVED FOOD GUIDELINES	LEVEL 2 APPROVED BEVERAGES
All naturally raised meats and fish	Filtered water	All naturally raised meats and fish	Filtered water
Eggs	Herbal tea (no caffeine)	Eggs**	Herbal tea (no caffeine)
Unsalted nuts	No-sugar- and no-fruit-added green juice	Unsalted nuts	No-sugar- and no-fruit-added green juice
Seeds	Coconut water	Seeds	Coconut water
Legumes (beans, peas, and lentils)	8 ounces of kombucha tea per day if desired	Legumes (beans, peas, and lentils)	8 ounces of kombucha tea per day if desired
All whole fruits	One cup of organic coffee per day if desired	All whole fruits	
All vegetables		All vegetables	
Organic corn	Green tea or matcha tea if desired		
Organic tofu or edamame			
Unsweetened Icelandic or Greek yogurt if taking this option			

**Eggs are a common allergen. If you've never eliminated them, consider eliminating them on your 28-day plan, then adding them back three times in one day to see how you feel. Some people feel great with eggs, and some feel worse. The only way to know is to test them by eliminating diligently for 28 days, then adding them back in. Remember to only add in one food every two days so if you have a reaction (e.g., headache, rash, low energy), you know which food causes it.

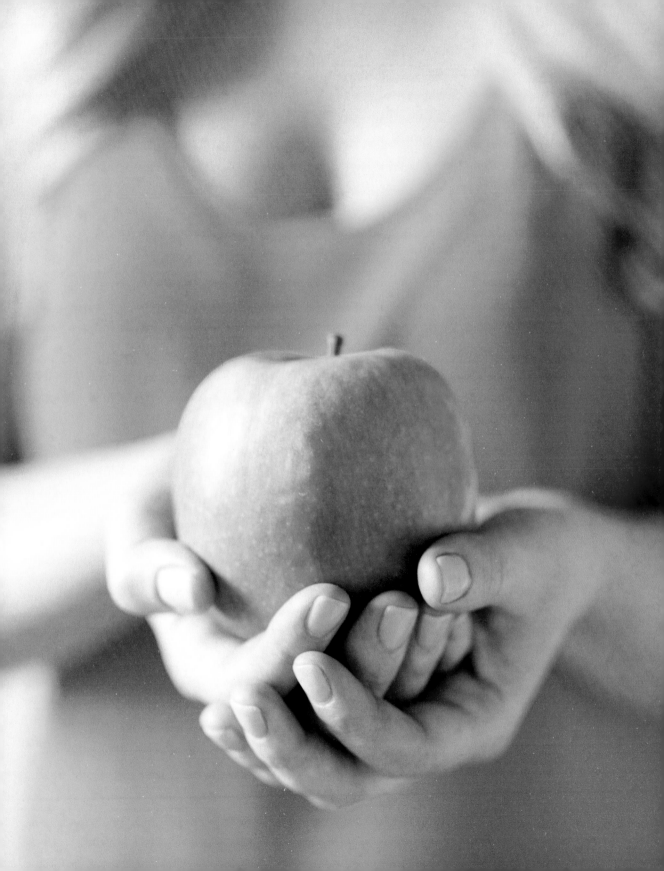

EXAMPLES OF *Approved* FOODS

Produce:

All whole fruits (no juices), fresh or frozen

Berries

Apples

Bananas

Melon

Citrus

All whole vegetables, fresh or frozen (either raw, steamed, sautéed, or roasted; no breading or frying)

Naturally raised meats:

Chicken

Turkey

Grass-fed beef

Nitrate-free deli meat

Salmon

Tuna

Halibut

*Eggs***:

Look for the highest-quality eggs that fit into your budget.

**See page 146.

Unsalted nuts:

Almonds

Walnuts

Pecans

Cashews

Brazil nuts

Pistachios

Macadamia nuts

Hazelnuts

Coconut:

Coconut juice, up to 12 ounces per day (no sugar added)

Fresh coconut "meat," if available

Coconut milk (look for cans of full-fat coconut, preferably in BPA-free cans)

Seeds:

Flaxseeds

Chia Seeds

Pumpkin seeds (aka pepitas)

Hemp seeds

Sunflower seeds

Quinoa (cooks like a grain, but technically a seed)

Legumes:

Black beans

Pinto beans

Chickpeas

Kidney beans

White beans

All types of peas

All colors of lentils

Organic peanuts*** (Level 1 only)

Organic tofu or edamame*** (Level 1 only)

Whole grains:

Whole rolled oats

Steel-cut oats

Rice

Millet

Organic corn*** (Level 1 only)

Other whole gluten-free grains you enjoy

***Items marked with three (***) are commonly genetically modified or stored in ways that allow mold to grow. Choose only organic if you choose to consume these options as organic varieties are non-GMO and generally stored in better conditions.

Oils and fats:

Extra-virgin olive oil

Flaxseed oil

Avocado oil

Virgin coconut oil, in moderation

Ghee (clarified butter in which the milk solids are removed)

Extras, condiments, and flavorings:

In general, check labels to ensure these items do not have added sugar.

All fermented veggies, such as kimchi or sauerkraut

Extra-virgin olive oil

Virgin coconut oil, in moderation

Apple cider vinegar

No-sugar-added salsa

No-sugar-added balsamic vinegar

Hot sauce (without preservatives)

Mustard

Tamari (wheat-free soy sauce; omit for Level 2)

Freshly squeezed lemon or lime juice, which adds wonderful flavor to your food and is an exception to the juice rule because it's low in sugar and high in nutrients

All spices, but read labels and nothing with fillers or preservatives

All fresh herbs

Unrefined sea salt, in moderation

Freshly ground coarse black pepper (because preground spices generally contain anticaking agents)

Portion sizes

In line with not asking you to count anything, I'm not going to ask you to weigh your food. However, be reasonable with portion sizes. It's okay to vary a little with these serving sizes; eat enough to feel full and stay mindful.

- One serving of cooked meat or fish is 3 ounces, which is about the side of a bar of soap or the palm of your hand. If you eat 4 ounces? Not a problem. A 16-ounce ribeye? That's too much—more than five times the amount of a serving.

- One serving of whole grains (oats, rice, quinoa) is ½ cup. That's about the size of your fist.

- One teaspoon of a healthy oil is the right serving size, which is about the side of your thumb to the first knuckle.

- One-fourth of a cup is a serving of nuts, while for nut butter, like almond butter, a serving is about 2 tablespoons.

- A serving of fruit is one small piece of whole fruit, or about ⅓ cup of berries or small fruits.

- Same goes for starchy veggies like potatoes, sweet potatoes, and beets. One-third of a cup is a serving.

- Eat as many green veggies and leafy greens as you'd like.

- Avocados get their own category because they're so special. One-half of a small avocado is a serving size, or about ¼ of a large one.

Eat local and in season

You can do this 28-day kick-start at any time of the year, and repeat it as often as you'd like. I give you loads of ideas here to get you started, and you'll want to adjust your meal plans to include in-season foods that make sense. You may not want to eat a hot soup in the summertime, so swap it out for a yummy fresh salad. If berries are expensive where you live, change them out for what's the best price at your store.

Success with this plan has more to do with planning ahead and coming up with ideas that you look forward to eating, and less to do with following my suggested meal plans and recipes exactly. If I suggest chicken but your store has a better deal on turkey, stay in the general guidelines and go for what fits for you.

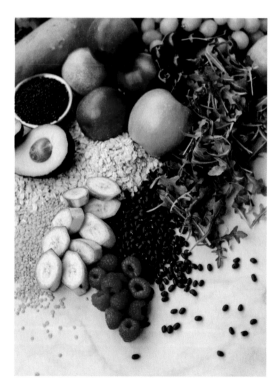

NOT-ALLOWED AT A GLANCE

THE NOT-ALLOWED LIST
Omit these items on your 28-day kick-start, and consider omitting them permanently after:

All added sugars, including white sugar or any other type of added sugar

Any type of processed meat

Anything with food coloring

Anything with gluten or wheat

Artificial sweeteners

Boxed cereal

Breaded meats

Canned fruit

Canned vegetables

Canola oil

Dairy (e.g., milk, cheese, cream, butter)

Dried fruits (except dates; see FAQ)

Fruit packed in juice or syrup

Highly processed grains

Juice

Preformed meat patties

Soda

Trans fats (look for the word *hydrogenated* in the ingredients list)

Vegetable oil

Wheat bread or noodles (even whole wheat)

APPROVED PACKAGED FOOD
These are not necessary, but they're okay to use on the program if desired:

Gluten-free rice noodles or gluten-free tortillas up to two times per week, if desired

Hot sauce without preservatives

Nitrate-free deli turkey or chicken

Rotisserie chicken (organic if possible) with the skin removed

Unsweetened, carrageenan-free nut milk

Unsweetened Icelandic or Greek yogurt if desired

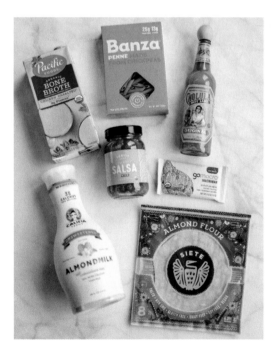

HEALTHY SUBSTITUTIONS CHART

INSTEAD OF THIS	TRY THIS
Bread crumbs	Whole rolled oats and/or nuts pulsed in a food processor
Conventional butter	Mashed avocado, extra virgin olive oil, virgin coconut oil (in moderation), macadamia nut oil, or ghee (clarified butter)
Conventional butter or vegetable oil in baked goods	Unsweetened apple sauce, mashed banana, or mashed avocado, depending on the recipe
Canned fruits and veggies	Fresh or frozen fruits and veggies
Chocolate chips	100% pure vegan dark chocolate chips
Conventional soy sauce	Organic tamari (wheat-free soy sauce) or coconut aminos
Couscous	Quinoa or cauliflower rice
Cow's milk	Unsweetened nut or seed milk (e.g., almond, walnut, or hemp milk); homemade is best, or look for carrageenen-free varieties
Cream cheese	Cashew cream cheese or almond cream cheese
Cream in savory soups	Pureed white beans, cashew cream, or coconut milk
Cream in sweet dishes	Coconut cream
Croutons	Toasted nuts or seeds
Eggs (in baking, if desired)	Make a vegan "flax egg" by mixing 1 tablespoon ground flax seeds with 3 tablespoons room-temperature water and letting sit for 15 minutes to gelatinize.
Ice cream	Dairy-free coconut milk ice cream or vegan banana "nice cream"
Instant oatmeal	Quinoa (serve it just like oats); steel-cut or old-fashioned oats
Mayonnaise	Homemade aioli or Vegenaise; plain unsweetened Greek yogurt; avocado puree

INSTEAD OF THIS	TRY THIS
Milk chocolate	Dark chocolate or raw chocolate (aka cacao)
Wheat or whole-wheat pasta	Quinoa or brown rice pasta
Pasta	Zucchini ribbons (zucchini shaved with a vegetable peeler); roasted spaghetti squash
Peanut butter	Almond or walnut butter
Pop/soda or other unhealthy drinks	Coconut water; kombucha; unsweetened tea; or club soda with fresh lemon or lime juice
Potato chips	Kale, sweet potato, or beet chips
Sour cream	Plain unsweetened Greek yogurt, chilled cashew cream, or chilled pureed avocado
Store-bought cereal	Homemade granola
Store-bought salad dressing	Homemade salad dressing or extra virgin olive oil and vinegar
Table salt	Real Salt brand sea salt, pink Himalayan salt, or Celtic Sea Salt
Tortillas or bread	Whole large romaine leaves or other greens
Vegetable oil	Extra virgin olive oil, virgin coconut oil, or macadamia nut oil (grapeseed oil is okay in moderation)
Wheat tortillas	Almond flour tortillas, rice flour tortillas, or lettuce wraps
White sugar	Raw honey, 100% real maple syrup, pitted dates (even natural sugars should be used in moderation after completing the 28-Day Kick-Start Plan)
Yogurt (sweetened/flavored)	Unsweetened plain Greek or Icelandic-style yogurt or Homemade Coconut Yogurt (page 188)

Kick-Start FAQS

Which is better, five small meals per day or three main meals with two small snacks?

This is one of most debated questions among health nuts around the world. In my opinion, it doesn't matter. Pick whatever works best for your lifestyle. Generally, the best plan is the one you will follow. If eating five small, same-size meals works for you and you feel energized, then do that. If you prefer three main meals (with or without small snacks), then do that. I don't think it's healthy over the long term to ask you to count calories or other food numbers, so I'm not going to ask you to do it in the kick-start. I've found that if you eat the way I've outlined here, you will naturally get the right amount of food.

The most important thing is to eat enough to satiate you until the next time you eat. When you do that without added sugars, your blood sugar will stabilize and you'll have enough energy throughout the day. If you have diabetes, please work with your health-care provider to determine the best option for you.

What about natural sweeteners like honey and maple syrup?

These things are A-OK to incorporate back in after the 28 days. During the 28-Day Kick-Start Plan, you're going to consume no-sugar-added foods to reset your taste buds and expectation of sweetness. While honey and maple are natural, they are still sources of added sugar. But don't fret! You can use whole fruits to sweeten your smoothies and sauces, and foods like roasted sweet potatoes, butternut squash, and carrots go a long way to adding a touch of sweetness to your meals.

This kick-start is going to reset your brain's expectation for sugar and sweetness; you'll be amazed at how much less you need when you add it back in.

Are dates allowed?

Dates (the dried fruit, not the boyfriend) are a great, whole, natural source of sugar and energy. I tend to group them in as an added natural sweetener with honey and maple, but I don't want to restrict you to the point that you cheat.

You're allowed up to two whole dates per day so you can still have some sweetness but not overload on the sugar. It's not necessary to eat them, but they'll help get you through if you have a sweet tooth. Blend a soaked, pitted date into a smoothie or sauce, or cut one in half and fill each side with almond butter for a kick-start treat. I like the Medjool variety.

What about stevia and monk fruit?

Just because they're all-natural, zero-calorie sweeteners doesn't mean that they can't set off a hormonal response in your body. Omit them during the 28 days and use them sparingly other times if desired.

My energy is dragging, what can I do?

It's normal to feel a decrease in energy during the first few days of a program like this. Keep up with the filtered water (60 to 70 ounces each day), and increase your veggie and whole-fruit intake for more energy. The good carbs in the veggies and whole fruit will give you more energy naturally.

I'm hungry, can I eat more?

Yes! Please do not starve yourself. Starving yourself slows your metabolism and no one wants to be hangry. Do a mindful check-in to see if you're hungry or just bored. Try some herbal tea or coconut water if you're simply looking for something with flavor. Add an extra meal or snack in line with the plan if you feel hungry.

What about restaurant food?

As I mentioned before, there is a wide span in the quality of food at restaurants. While it's true that there are some small local restaurants that you can count on to tell the truth and where everything is prepared in-house, the real truth is that the majority of restaurant food is not prepared in the restaurant, even at nice places. Even if they do prepare the foods, they most likely use condiments and sauces that contain lower-quality oils like canola or vegetable oil.

In an ideal world, you would eat only food you prepare yourself during these 28 days. If that's not realistic, try to prepare as much of your own food as possible, and stick to the guidelines when dining out or traveling. In some cities there are fresh and healthy restaurants that make food in line with these guidelines. Still ask about ingredients of dressings and sauces, and if they fit into the guidelines and you can afford to dine out then feel free to incorporate them.

The bottom line is that the food needs to fit into what's acceptable in the kick-start.

What about chocolate? (aka Woman, I need chocolate!)

Like I said before, I'm not a monster. One square of at least 70 percent cocoa high-quality vegan dark chocolate is allowed each day if you need your fix.

Will I lose weight on this kick-start?

If you have excess weight to lose, then you will most likely lose weight on this plan. If weight loss is your specific goal, eliminate all grains after 3 P.M. and aim for a 14- to 16-hour fasting window between dinner and breakfast the next morning. If you need to review, fasting windows are discussed with time-restricted eating in Chapter 3.

Can I modify this kick-start?

You'll get the best results if you stick to the 28-Day Kick-Start Plan as designed. If you feel you need to modify it, only give up one thing at a time, like gluten or added sugars.

Whoopsies, I cheated. Now what?

Get right back on the horse! All of your efforts are not for nothing. Make your absolute best effort not to cheat, but if you do, pick up immediately where you left off. Also, understand the cheat trigger. Were you too hungry because you didn't eat enough in your last meal? Was it an emotional trigger? Try to understand what happened so you can be prepared.

MORE MEAL AND SNACK IDEAS

Feel free to mix and match these to fit your tastes:

BREAKFAST	LUNCH OR DINNER	SNACKS
2 scrambled eggs with black beans and hot sauce, if desired	Anything from the breakfast category, because who doesn't love breakfast for dinner?	1 piece of whole fruit with 1 to 2 tablespoons unsweetened nut butter
1 whole egg plus 1 or 2 egg whites with sautéed spinach, black beans, and hot sauce	Roasted chicken or turkey breast or fish with roasted veggies of your choice	Unsweetened Icelandic or Greek yogurt with ¼ cup fruit of your choice, sprinkled with chia seeds
2 scrambled eggs with sautéed spinach and ½ cup roasted sweet potato	Tuna salad or chicken salad in lettuce cups	Hummus with veggies
Green Beauty Smoothie (see recipe, page 169)	Healthy Slow-Cooker Chicken Tacos (see recipe, page 232)	½ small avocado with cherry tomatoes, drizzled with 1 teaspoon extra-virgin olive oil and ½ teaspoon balsamic vinegar
Sweet Berry Smoothie (see recipe, page 168)	Game-Day Chili (see recipe, page 234)	1 to 2 hard-boiled eggs with salt and pepper
"Cake Batter" Smoothie (see recipe, page 169)	Hummus, Quinoa & Superfood Veggie Bowl (see recipe at www.elizabethrider.com)	¼ cup coconut milk and ½ cup water blended with ½ cup frozen fruit and 2 soaked, pitted dates
Coconut milk smoothie with ½ cup coconut milk, 1 cup filtered water, ½ avocado, and ½ cup fruit	Spaghetti Squash "Noodles" (see recipe, page 199) with your favorite sauce	10 ounces of bone broth
2-Ingredient Egg & Banana Pancakes (see recipe, page 174)	Easy Lentil Soup (see recipe, page 214)	Homemade guacamole with veggie sticks
Hemp & Chia Seed Overnight Oats (see recipe, page 176)	Homemade Thai Red Curry (see recipe, page 226) over veggies and quinoa	½ cup overnight oats with apple slices or berries
Reimagined Hashbrown Casserole (see recipe, page 182)	Black Bean & Sweet Potato Superfood Salad (see recipe, page 208) with chicken if desired	½ cup chia seed pudding
Unsweetened Icelandic or Greek yogurt with ½ cup fruit of your choice, sprinkled with chia seeds	Any of the soups from my website or in this book	Olives with mixed veggies
Quinoa with nut milk, warmed on the stove like oatmeal and topped with fruit	Any of the smoothies from my website or in this book	½ portion of anything on the meal lists

OMG, I'm Underprepared and Need Something Now!

Try not to rely on these because it's impossible to be sure what's in them, but if you're in a pinch and need to grab and go or must dine out, here are some acceptable things that will keep you on track:

- Pho soup from a Vietnamese restaurant, but only if they don't use MSG.

- Good-quality sushi. Look for fish with rice and veggies. Ask for extra avocado and avoid saucy things.

- Build-your-own salad at the grocery store salad bar.

- A nut-based, low-sugar nutrition bar. There are literally thousands on the market so I can't recommend a specific brand, but if you can find one with less than 10 grams of sugar and you're in a pinch it's okay. Don't rely on them as a mainstay.

#1 Morning Hydration

Upon rising, hydrate before anything else. Just like you can fog a mirror with your breath, you lose a lot of moisture while you sleep simply from breathing. Drinking 20 to 30 ounces of filtered water first thing in the morning rehydrates your body with moisture lost during sleep. You'll find you're less hungry during the day and your skin looks more hydrated when you start the day off this way.

If you love hot water with freshly squeezed lemon juice in the morning, you can do that instead—or do both. Breaking your overnight fast with this jump-starts your digestion and provides a big boost of alkalizing vitamin C.

If you're not into that, it's okay, but do make a habit of drinking those 20 to 30 ounces first thing. I place my glass water bottle next to my bed at night so it's ready for me first thing. In the morning, after your lemon water, consider a fasted workout to burn even more fat.

#2 Jump-Start Your Digestion

Ten to 20 minutes before breakfast, consider a simple shot of apple cider vinegar or fresh lemon juice. Dilute it slightly with filtered water so the taste is easier to take (and to protect your tooth enamel). One tablespoon apple cider vinegar or fresh lemon juice to two tablespoons filtered water works great. Or, dilute it even more in a big mug of hot (but not boiling!) water like the lemon water I mentioned above.

Lemon juice and apple cider vinegar are naturally acidic before you consume them, but create an alkaline environment in your digestive system to optimize digestion and boost your metabolism. They also kick your digestive enzymes into gear, prepping your body to break your overnight fast. Add a few grates of fresh ginger for an even bigger health boost.

#3 Breaking Your Fast

As you learned in Chapter 6, what you eat first thing in the morning sets the tone for your entire day. Commit to only low-glycemic food when you break your overnight fast (breakfast) to keep your blood sugar stable and prevent hunger, cravings, and anxiety.

This meal will also start the clock on your eating window if you're following an intermittent fasting schedule. If weight loss is your goal, be sure to consume 20 to 30 grams of protein in your first meal of the day.

EXAMPLES: low-glycemic smoothie; 2 eggs with sautéed greens plus ¼ roasted sweet potato; superfood overnight oats; 2-Ingredient Egg and Banana Pancakes (see recipe, page 174); or a slice of Flexible Veggie Frittata (see recipe, page 184).

Enjoy a cup of organic coffee with almond milk (no sugar added), green tea, or herbal tea before, after, or with your breakfast if you'd like.

#4 Snacks

Snacks can fuel you up and help you get through the day. I find it's a personal choice; some people are snackers and some are not. I like to include a midmorning and midafternoon snack to keep my energy up and metabolism humming.

If you choose not to snack, because you're busy or forget, then be sure to eat enough at each meal to fuel your energy until your next meal. If you let yourself go hungry you're more likely to overeat. Snacks should stick to the same guiding principles we've already discussed. Low-sugar, minimally processed options are always best.

EXAMPLES: handful of nuts; chia seed pudding; homemade energy bites; an 8 ounce-sugar smoothie; a mug of bone broth; veggie sticks with hummus; a hard-boiled egg with veggies; ½ avocado sprinkled with sea salt; a slice of almond flour bread; or whole fruit with almond butter.

#5 Lunch

Combine a healthy protein, good fat, and good carbohydrate for a balanced lunch that will fuel you for the rest of the day.

#6 Dinner

Choose from lean proteins, good fats, and bigger portions of greens or vegetables than grains.

EXAMPLES: a big salad with chicken or salmon; coconut milk-based veggie curry with brown rice or quinoa; chicken tacos in lettuce wraps; broiled fish with greens and veggies; a hearty soup or chili; or a healthy stir-fry.

If you're a wine drinker, one glass of high-quality wine a few nights a week after the kick-start is absolutely acceptable. Choose drier varieties to limit added sugars.

#7 After Dinner

Herbal tea is always a wonderful after-dinner option. Peppermint tea, in particular, has been used for centuries to aid digestion. Studies have shown that it helps relieve gas and bloating, and can reduce heartburn and indigestion as well. It also tastes and smells delightful. Ending your meal with peppermint tea hits the sweet spot without adding any extra sugar to your meal. It's zero-calorie, naturally caffeine-free, and doesn't contain any sugar.

Many of my clients find this post-dinner habit replaces cravings for sugary desserts. If you're a dessert lover, a small, raw, low-sugar dessert within an hour after dinner is A-OK. Look for something made from whole foods.

#8 Start Your Fasting Window

Be sure to eat a large, healthful, low-glycemic meal at dinner to balance your blood sugar and provide enough energy until morning. If you're new to this approach, a 10-hour eating window (e.g., 8 A.M. to 6 P.M. or 9 A.M. to 7 P.M.) is a good start. That means you fast from after dinner at 7 p.m. until 9 a.m. the next day.

Review the concept of your fasting window in Chapter 3 if needed. Giving your insulin levels a break will help you feel better, have increased energy, and more easily manage your weight.

#9 Prepare for Tomorrow

Remember, failing to plan is planning to fail. Take a few minutes to think about what needs to happen tomorrow. If you need to prep any delicious meals or snacks to have on hand, do that now, then cozy up with a big hot mug of tea or a good book and relax. You deserve it.

Sample Meal Plans (ADJUST ACCORDINGLY)

SAMPLE Day 1

7 A.M.	Morning hydration
8 A.M.	"Cake Batter" Smoothie (see recipe, page 169) + supplements
10:30 A.M.	Hard-boiled egg with carrots & hummus
12:30 P.M.	Easy Lentil Soup (see recipe, page 214)
3 P.M.	½ apple with 2 tablespoons almond butter
6 P.M.	Healthy Slow-Cooker Chicken Tacos (see recipe, page 232)
7 P.M.	Peppermint tea (optional: with a square of dark chocolate)

SAMPLE Day 2

7 A.M.	Morning hydration
8 A.M.	2 scrambled eggs with black beans + supplements
10:30 A.M.	½ cup overnight oats with berries
12:30 P.M.	Tuna salad in lettuce cups
3 P.M.	Tropical Coconut Smoothie (see recipe, page 168)
6 P.M.	Roasted chicken with asparagus and roasted butternut squash
7 P.M.	8 ounces coconut water or tea

SAMPLE Day 3

7 A.M.	Morning hydration
8 A.M.	2-Ingredient Egg & Banana Pancakes (see recipe, page 174) without syrup + supplements
10:30 A.M.	Greek or coconut yogurt with ½ cup fruit of your choice
12:30 P.M.	Dairy-free cashew pesto over penne rice noodles
3 P.M.	Green Beauty Smoothie (see recipe, page 169)
6 P.M.	Game-Day Chili (see recipe, page 234) with guacamole
7 P.M.	No-Bake Extra Chocolatey Chocolate Avocado Mousse (see recipe, page 236)

SAMPLE *Day 4*

7 A.M.	Morning hydration
8 A.M.	Black beans with salsa and ½ avocado + supplements
10:30 A.M.	1 date, split in half, each half stuffed with ½ tablespoon nut butter
12:30 P.M.	Black Bean and Sweet Potato Superfood Salad (see recipe, page 208)
3 P.M.	Chocolate protein smoothie
6 P.M.	10-Minute Maple Dijon Salmon (see salmon recipe, page 231)
7 P.M.	Mint tea

SAMPLE *Day 5*

7 A.M.	Morning hydration
8 A.M.	Sweet Berry Smoothie (see recipe, page 168) + supplements
10:30 A.M.	1 date, split in half, each half stuffed with ½ tablespoon of nut butter
12:30 P.M.	Loaded veggie & avocado lettuce wraps
3 P.M.	Black Bean & Quinoa Salad (see recipe, page 207)
6 P.M.	Homemade bunless burgers with Baked Sweet Potato Fries (see recipe, page 196)
7 P.M.	Mint tea

SAMPLE *Day 6*

7 A.M.	Morning hydration
8 A.M.	"Cake Batter" Smoothie (see recipe, page 169) + supplements
10:30 A.M.	1 slice Almond Flour Bread with Stove-Top Chia Seed Jam (see recipes, pages 190 and 191)
12:30 P.M.	Easy Lentil Soup (see recipe, page 214)
3 P.M.	Greek or Homemade Coconut Yogurt (see recipe, page 188) with ½ cup fruit of your choice
6 P.M.	Homemade Thai Red Curry (see recipe, page 226)
7 P.M.	Peppermint tea (optional: with a square of dark chocolate)

7 A.M.	Morning hydration
8 A.M.	2 scrambled eggs on a gluten-free tortilla with hot sauce + supplements
10:30 A.M.	Greek or Homemade Coconut Yogurt (see recipe, page 188) with ½ cup fruit of your choice
12:30 P.M.	Big mixed-veggie salad with Healthy Honey Mustard Dressing (see recipe, page 202)
3 P.M.	½ cup overnight oats with berries
6 P.M.	Roasted chicken with Magic Sauce (see recipe, page 192) and green beans
7 P.M.	Peppermint tea (optional: with a square of dark chocolate)

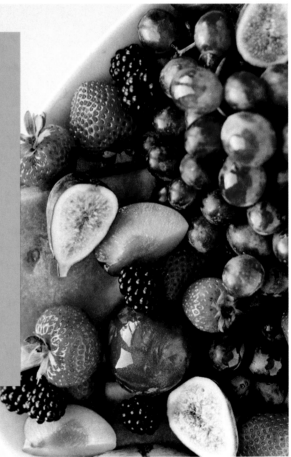

What's Your Eating Style?

Before you begin this program, get acquainted with the 28-Day Kick-Start Plan's eating guidelines. Determine if you're a *moderator*, an *abstainer*, or a mix of the two to help guide your food choices (see page 36 for a refresher on these terms). Make a list of your top 10 favorite meals and snacks that fit into these guidelines and/or the eating style that you choose. Make a shopping list based on the top 10 favorite meals and snacks and head to the store to stock up on what you need.

DAY BY DAY ON THE
28-DAY KICK-START PLAN

One small change per day can add up to huge results. To keep you motivated, I'm giving you 28 daily prompts to up your health game during your kick-start. If you want to do a few on the same day, that works. Or, if you want to switch things around, that works too. If you're not ready to replace everything at the same time, just move toward healthy options as you run out of things and need to substitute. If I could, I'd add getting "Consistency Beats Perfection" tattooed on your forehead as one of your daily actions, but I've heard tattoos can be expensive and I want to stay in your budget. Do your absolute best to stick to the food guidelines and try not to cheat, because if you cheat on the food you're cheating yourself out of knowing how gluten, dairy, and added sugar affects you. You deserve to know the truth. Stick to the plan but remember your original goal of progress and consistency, not perfection.

The day before you start, please get a journal or grab a dedicated notebook to be your kick-start journal. Take a moment to handwrite your goals for this 28-Day Kick-Start Plan. I outlined how to do this in Chapter 1. If you need a refresher, use these prompts in order:

1. What is your desired outcome?

2. Why?

3. How would this make you feel?

4. What outcome would support the feeling you just identified that you desire?

5. What daily actionable steps will get you there?

Here is an example:

1. **What is your desired outcome?**

   I want to have more energy in the morning while I'm with my kids.

2. **Why?**

   We all have more fun when I have more energy, and I want to enjoy my mornings more.

3. **How would this make you feel?**

   This would make me feel more productive, more connected to my kids, more joyful in daily life.

4. **What outcome would support the feeling you just identified that you desire?**

   If I could get to a point of going to bed before 9:30 p.m. so I can be asleep by 10, I could get eight hours of uninterrupted sleep.

5. **What daily actionable steps will get you there?**

   My daily actionable steps would be: to eat a low-glycemic dinner, not have any sugar or alcohol after 6 p.m., and create a nighttime routine that gets me excited for bed.

28-Day Kick-Start Plan

DAY 0 (THE DAY(S) BEFORE): Consider your eating style, choose your meals from the meal plan, and make your shopping list. Journal your goals for the plan.

DAY 1: Start today! Eat according to the kick-start guidelines today and continue on for 28 days. Prepare meals as needed on the program.

DAY 2: Commit to morning hydration—20 to 30 ounces of filtered water first thing in the morning, before anything else, every day, to rehydrate your body from moisture lost while sleeping.

DAY 3: Batch-prepare at least three days' worth of lunches.

DAY 4: Write out your morning self-care routine and start to stick to it. Try it out for a few mornings in a row. How does it feel? Does something need to be adjusted?

DAY 5: Write out your evening self-care routine and start to stick to it. Try it out for a few evenings in a row. How does it feel? Does something need to be adjusted?

DAY 6: Schedule your exercise into your calendar now for the next month. Five days of at least 30 minutes of activity is the baseline. It can be anything from a morning or pre-breakfast walk, to an exercise class, hike, run, yoga, or your favorite heart-pumping activity. Consider it an appointment with yourself that you cannot miss.

DAY 7: Check the house for triclosan-containing ingredients and dispose of or donate them.

DAY 8: Buy yourself some fresh flowers or a new plant to liven up your kitchen or living room. Finding pleasure and joy outside of food is a key element to success.

DAY 9: Get outside today. Take some time to simply enjoy being outdoors and feel gratitude for nature.

DAY 10: Take a breather and give yourself 10 or 15 minutes to meditate or sit in quietness and observe your breath. Add this to your daily schedule going forward as part of your new Health Habit.

DAY 11: Measure your waist and record it to compare to the end of the kick-start and six months from now. You can also do this on Day 1 and Day 28 of your kick-start to track your results.

DAY 12: Try a new recipe today that fits in the guidelines of the kick-start.

DAY 13: Acquire and start reading an uplifting book. I suggest *The Alchemist* by Paulo Coelho if you haven't read it, or *The Four Agreements* by Don Miguel Ruiz as it will change your life. Grab one from your local library, a friend, or any bookstore.

DAY 14: Reevaluate your bedtime routine and the use of blue-light-emitting electronics before bed. Is there anywhere for improvement here?

DAY 15: Make your appointment for your annual well-woman exam and physical.

DAY 16: Healthy kitchen check-in: Toss plastic utensils and make a plan to replace items discussed in Chapter 5 now or as you are able.

DAY 17: Indulge in a hot bath with Epsom salts and essential oils, or other healthy spa-like treatment you desire.

DAY 18: Laundry check-in: Read ingredient labels and make a plan to replace items such as your laundry detergent now or as you are able.

DAY 19: Try this brilliant happiness trick from Google pioneer Chade-Meng Tan to experience "the joy of loving-kindness." Randomly identify two people (either in the room you're in, or whom you've recently encountered) and think, *I wish for this person to be happy, and I wish for this person to be happy.* As a bonus, continue to do this throughout the day, and/or add this to your morning gratitude routine. Enjoy the wave of happiness from wishing others to be happy.

DAY 20: Beauty products check-in: You guessed it, read ingredient labels and make a plan to replace items now or as you are able.

DAY 21: Today, try something new, like a type of tea, wellness therapy, or food that you've been wanting to try (and that fits in our guidelines, of course).

DAY 22: Period care check-in (if needed): Evaluate what the healthiest option is for you and follow it.

DAY 23: Recommit to your water habits and drink half your body weight in ounces today. Bonus if you're already doing that and want to add a no-sugar-added green juice to your daily meal plan.

DAY 24: Schedule an active date with a friend, like hiking, a long walk, or visiting a museum.

DAY 25: Now that you're getting the swing of eating this way, write out a Monday-through-Friday meal plan that fits into these guidelines and works for you. Use this five-day meal plan starting next week.

DAY 26: Time to reflect. Use the journal prompt exercises at the end of Chapter 7 and spend at least one hour (total) answering the questions related to the Intangibles.

DAY 27: Yesterday was probably intense, so take a breather and give yourself 10 or 15 minutes to meditate or sit in quietness and observe your breath. Continue to journal to get your thoughts onto paper so new thoughts and feelings can emerge.

DAY 28: Celebrate! Toast yourself with a glass of kombucha or tea (you're not done yet) and grab your journal. Write out everything you think and feel about this 28-day experience. What were the best parts? What was the most difficult? What will you continue to commit to? What advice would you give your past self? What advice would you give your future self?

**GET YOUR FREE PRINTABLE
28-DAY PROGRAM TRACKER AT
ELIZABETHRIDER.COM/BOOK
TO FOLLOW ALONG.**

Cashew Basil Mint Pesto, p. 195

CHAPTER 10

Health Habit Recipes

Easy Recipes to Support a Healthier You

L et's eat! Now that you're all schooled up on healthier habits, it's time to enjoy the flavors and nutritional benefits of some delightfully easy recipes. Here you'll find a sampling of the most popular recipes from my blog, along with some client favorites and a few that are brand new just for this book.

The selection here is a mere sampling of the endless healthy whole food meals and snacks available to create. I mentioned back in Chapter 3 that I don't label my eating habits, so you'll notice that these don't fall into the exact same categories. I have, however, added a few dietary labels for quick identification for those who need them.

We had room for 50 recipes here, but head on over to my website (elizabethrider.com) for dozens more.

Protein Powder

Check that the protein powder is dairy-free, if desired. There are a variety of protein powders available. Whey protein comes from milk and works for some people who tolerate dairy. Pea protein and hemp protein are dairy-free, vegan sources of protein.

TROPICAL COCONUT SMOOTHIE

If you'd like to transport yourself to a warmer, sunnier climate, this smoothie will help do the trick. It's nutritious and delicious—and you'll feel like you're lounging on a beach in the Bahamas. Not a bad deal for a smoothie!

———

MAKES 1 SERVING

Gluten-Free, Dairy-Free, Vegan

———

½ cup full-fat coconut milk (from a can, not a carton)

½ cup fresh or frozen pineapple (not canned)

1 cup filtered water

Ice

½ avocado

Blend all the ingredients and enjoy immediately.

SWEET BERRY SMOOTHIE

There are antioxidants and polyphenols galore in this balanced smoothie of low-glycemic berries, protein, healthy fats from nuts and seeds, and just a bit of sweetness from a banana. Voilà! The perfect quick meal.

———

MAKES 1 SERVING

Gluten-Free, Dairy-Free

———

1 serving high-quality protein powder (see sidebar page 167)

1 teaspoon seeds or nuts

12 to 16 ounces filtered water

½ cup fresh or frozen berries of your choice

1 serving collagen powder, optional

1 small frozen banana

Blend all the ingredients and enjoy immediately.

GREEN BEAUTY SMOOTHIE

Get your daily dose of leafy greens with this healthy and delicious smoothie. Collagen powder helps keep your skin firm and your hair and nails long and strong. It's not vegan, so omit if you prefer a vegan smoothie.

————

MAKES 1 SERVING

Gluten-Free, Dairy-Free

————

1 serving high-quality vanilla protein powder (see sidebar page 167)

1 handful of fresh greens

1 small frozen banana

1 teaspoon seeds or nuts

12 to 16 ounces filtered water

1 serving collagen powder, optional

Blend all the ingredients and enjoy immediately.

"CAKE BATTER" SMOOTHIE

This smoothie sounds heavenly and even a little sinful, I know—but rest assured, it's all health coach-approved. And it's actually healthy, too.

————

MAKES 1 SERVING

Gluten-Free, Dairy-Free, Vegan

————

1 serving high-quality protein powder (see sidebar page 167)

1 small frozen banana

2 teaspoons unsweetened almond butter

¼ teaspoon high-quality vanilla extract

1 small pinch of sea salt

12 to 16 ounces filtered water

1 soaked, pitted date for extra sweetness, optional

Blend all the ingredients and enjoy immediately.

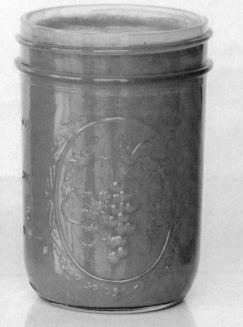

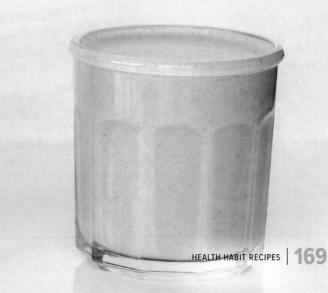

HEALTHY HOMEMADE COFFEE CREAMER

This recipe is dairy-free, gluten-free, and of course way healthier than the store-bought version, which usually includes casein, sugar, sodium, and corn syrup (yuck!). This homemade option ensures you'll have a nutritious and healthy creamer, and for less money, too.

MAKES 2 CUPS

Gluten-Free, Dairy-Free, Vegan option

½ **cup raw cashews, soaked for 12 hours**

1½ **cups filtered water**

Pinch of sea salt

2 **teaspoons maple syrup (vegan) or manuka honey (not vegan)**

¼ **teaspoon cinnamon**

¼ **teaspoon vanilla (more or less to taste)**

Drain and rinse the cashews. Blend all the ingredients on high in a high-speed blender until smooth. Store for up to 1 week in the refrigerator.

NOTE: You can choose to soak your cashew nuts overnight at room temp, or you can do a quick soak in hot (but not boiling) water for 1 hour.

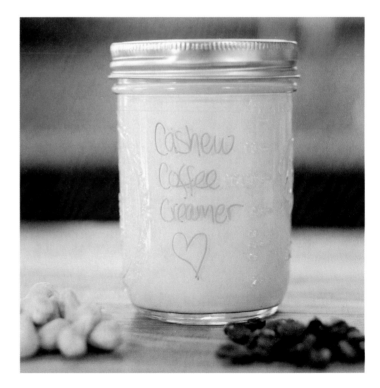

GOLDEN MILK
(AKA TURMERIC TEA)

If you haven't tried golden milk (aka turmeric tea or turmeric latte), then now is the perfect time to whip up a batch. This traditional Ayurvedic drink is nourishing and smooth, and it's quite simple to make. The pinch of black pepper helps your body better absorb all the anti-inflammatory elements in the turmeric. Enjoy any time of day.

MAKES 2 SERVINGS

Gluten-Free, Dairy-Free, Vegan option

1 cup unsweetened almond milk

1 to 2 teaspoons almond oil

½ teaspoon ground turmeric

Big pinch of freshly ground black pepper

1 small (¼-inch) piece of ginger root, peeled and grated

Big pinch of ground cardamom

¼ teaspoon raw honey (not vegan) or maple syrup (vegan) added off the heat, optional

Blend all the ingredients, then warm on the stove. Simmer (do not boil) for 15 minutes. You can blend the ingredients by hand or in a high-speed blender for a frothier drink.

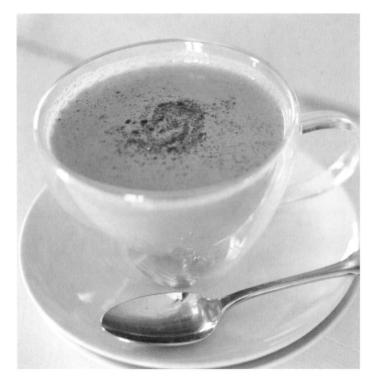

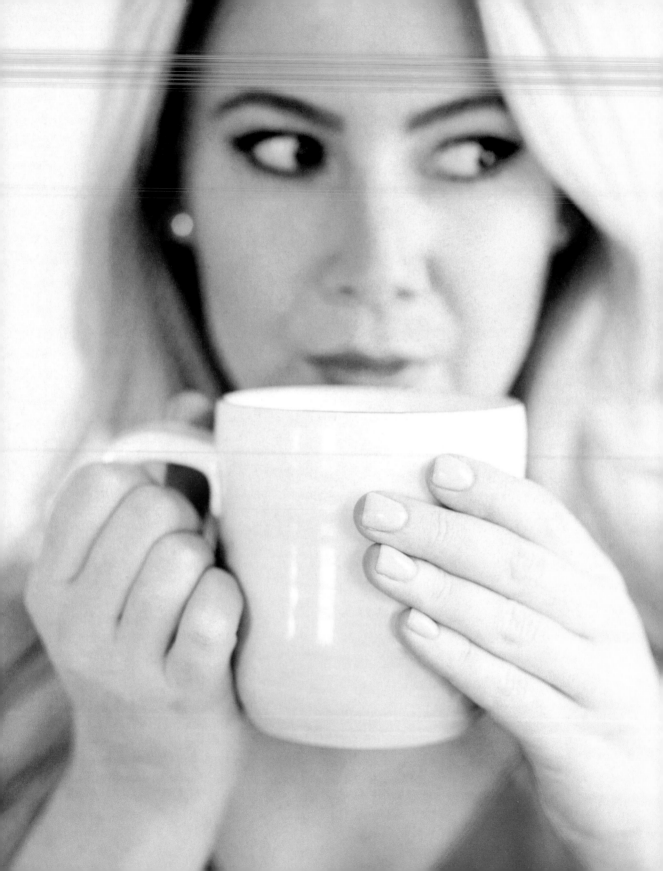

"MAKE ME SLEEPY" ELIXIR

Try this simple natural concoction for a more restful night's sleep. Honey has been used for centuries as a sleep aid. Choose raw honey as it will have more enzymes and be less processed. Hot water will kill some of the enzymes in both the honey and apple cider vinegar, but it doesn't ruin all of their nutritional benefits (this is why we use hot, not boiling, water). For this recipe, I boil water in my electric kettle and let it sit for 5 to 10 minutes before using. There aren't any scientific studies as to why this nighttime drink works, but it does. Some nutrition experts hypothesize that raw honey replenishes liver glycogen more efficiently than anything else, which allows you to stay asleep longer. Try not to drink so much liquid that it wakes you up in the middle of the night, which disrupts your good night's sleep.

MAKES 1 SERVING

Gluten-Free, Dairy-Free, Vegan option

1 tablespoon raw honey (I prefer manuka)

1 tablespoon apple cider vinegar

8 to 12 ounces of hot (but not boiling) filtered water

1 tea bag made for sleep, optional

Boil the water, then let it sit for about five minutes. Mix in the rest of the ingredients and enjoy about 1 hour before bedtime. The honey and apple cider vinegar alone does the trick for most people. Add 1 bag of sleep-inducing tea from a trusted brand for nights when you need even more help.

2-INGREDIENT EGG & BANANA PANCAKES

You can make healthy and delicious pancakes with just banana, egg, and a little healthy oil (I use coconut oil) for the cast-iron pan. A cast-iron pan over medium heat is best for this; trust me, I've made many a batch of egg and banana pancakes that won't flip or stick to the pan. I also like to boost up the flavor with a high-quality vanilla extract and cinnamon.

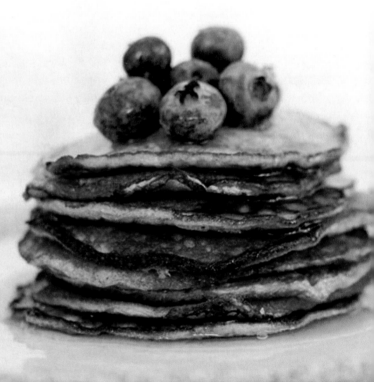

MAKES 2 SERVINGS (2 TO 3 SMALL PANCAKES EACH)

Gluten-Free, Dairy-Free

1 medium to large ripe banana*

2 large eggs

⅛ teaspoon sea salt, optional

¼ teaspoon pure vanilla extract, optional

¼ teaspoon cinnamon, optional

½ teaspoon coconut oil (for cooking)

*Proportions can vary, but in general, a medium to large banana and 2 large (not extra-large or jumbo) eggs work. If you have a small banana and a jumbo egg, just use 1 of each. One banana and 2 eggs will give you about 5 or maybe 6 pancakes when you use a ¼-cup measuring cup.

Preheat a cast-iron pan over medium heat for 10 minutes. A nice medium heat is important: If the pan is too hot, the pancakes will burn; if it's not hot enough, they won't set. If you have a newer/professional-style gas stove top, start with medium-low heat, because those puppies have more power than a standard stove top.

While the pan preheats, mix the ingredients into a smooth batter. I use a hand mixer because I find it easy, but you can use a blender, mixer, or do it by hand by mashing the banana really well then mixing in your other ingredients. Regardless of the method, mix the batter until it's well-combined, about 30 to 60 seconds, but don't whip too much air into it (eggs will eventually whip up into foam if you let it go too long).

Add about ½ teaspoon coconut oil to the pan and spread it around with your spatula right before you add the batter. Don't preheat the oil with the pan because it will get too hot. Grapeseed oil or macadamia nut oil can work too, but extra-virgin olive oil doesn't have a high enough smoke point and will smoke too much. Coconut oil is healthy, can withstand high heat, and adds a very light, yummy flavor to the pancakes, so it's my oil of choice here.

Using a ¼-cup measuring cup, add your batter to the pan right after the coconut oil is melted (that only takes about 10 seconds). Important: Set your kitchen timer for 2 minutes. I cook them on the first side for 2 minutes to allow them to set properly. Check them at 1 minute 45 seconds, but don't try to flip them too early. Once you get the hang of it, you'll know when to flip.

Once the pancakes are set (again, about 2 minutes—give or take 10 to 15 seconds), use a spatula big enough to get under the entire pancake and flip them over. Cook another 1 ½ minutes (give or take 10 to 15 seconds) for the perfect 2-ingredient pancake.

Stack 'em up! If you want, drizzle the top with 1 tablespoon raw honey, pure maple syrup, and ½ cup berries, or maple cashew cream.

HEMP & CHIA SEED OVERNIGHT OATS

Preparing overnight oats is as simple as pouring nut milk over a few ingredients. Healthy eating doesn't get any easier than this. And, it's delicious (of course). This recipe will become a staple in your healthy kitchen in no time.

MAKES 1 SERVING

Gluten-Free, Dairy-Free, Vegan option

½ cup whole rolled oats, preferably organic

2 teaspoons chia seeds

2 teaspoons hemp seeds (aka hemp hearts)

1 tablespoon unsweetened coconut flakes, optional

½ cup unsweetened almond milk or other nondairy milk of your choice

About ⅓ cup fresh or frozen berries (for topping)

Drizzle of raw honey (not vegan) or maple syrup (vegan) for flavor, nutrients, and natural sweetness, optional

Mix the oats, chia seeds, and hemp seeds in a small bowl or jar (I use 8-ounce containers). Top with the unsweetened coconut flakes, if using. Pour the nut milk over the oat mixture—it should be saturated to the point where the milk pools on top a little. Cover and refrigerate overnight, or up to 3 days. Top with berries and/or a small drizzle of raw honey or maple syrup before eating, if using.

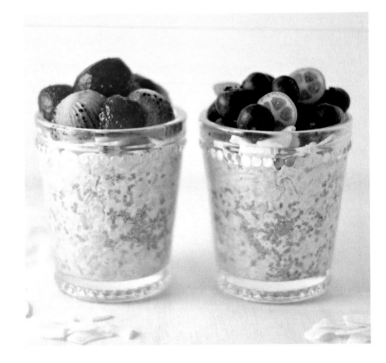

QUINOA BERRY BREAKFAST BOWL

A seed that cooks like a grain, cooked quinoa is one of the most versatile ingredients in your kitchen. It makes a great substitute for cooked rice or grains in just about any savory dish, but you might not know that it's great in sweet preparations, too. This breakfast bowl makes a great, simple, healthy breakfast when you're trying to avoid grains and/or boost your protein intake in the morning.

MAKES 1 SERVING

Gluten-Free, Dairy-Free, Vegan

½ cup cooked quinoa

Sprinkle of cinnamon

Nondairy milk of your choice, such as almond milk, oat milk, or cashew milk

⅓ cup berries

1 teaspoon chia seeds, flaxseeds, or hemp seeds (or a combo of all 3)

1 teaspoon of raw honey or maple syrup, optional

Place the quinoa in a bowl, sprinkle with cinnamon, then top with nondairy milk. Add the berries, sprinkle the seeds over, and top with honey or syrup, if desired. Enjoy.

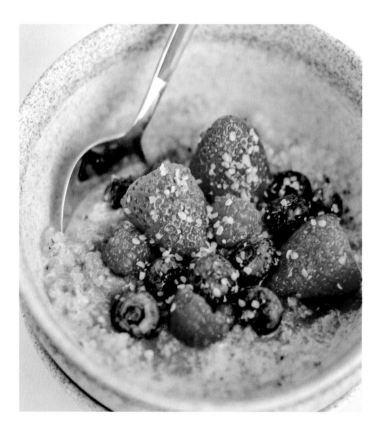

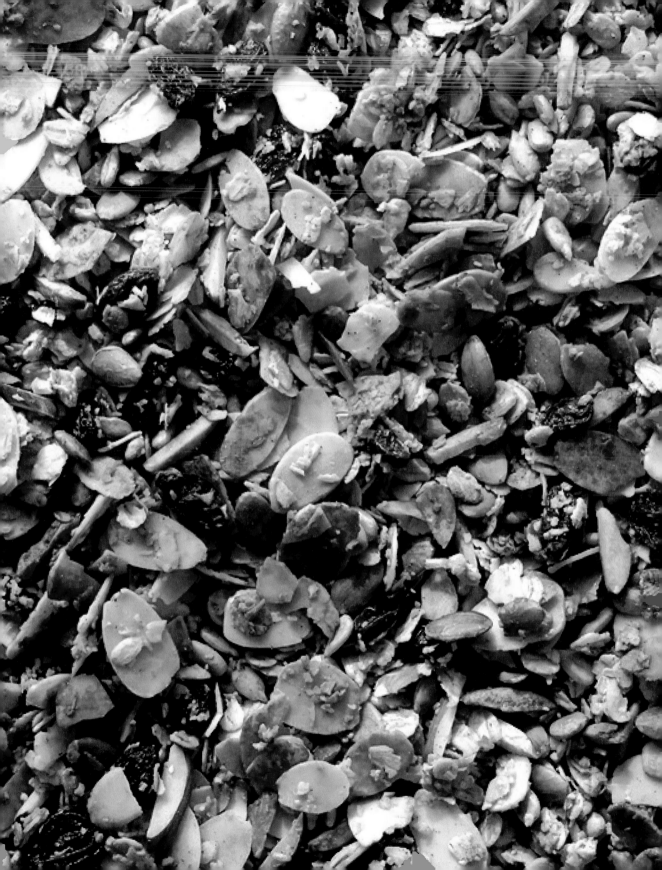

HEALTHY HOMEMADE GRANOLA

Homemade granola can be a healthy, comforting, and delicious treat. Whipping up your own at home is super easy and quick. Homemade granola also makes your house smell amazing—like you've been slaving in the kitchen all day. This is the number-one homemade granola recipe on Google for good reason. It's delicious, simple, and definitely healthier than store-bought granola.

MAKES 3 CUPS (ABOUT 6 ½-CUP SERVINGS)

Gluten-Free, Dairy-Free, Vegan

2 cups raw whole rolled oats* (aka old-fashioned oats), preferably organic

½ cup raw nuts, chopped

¼ cup raw seeds (sunflower or pumpkin seeds are great)

½ cup unsweetened dried fruit, chopped, optional

2 to 3 tablespoons maple syrup (vegan) or raw honey (not vegan), or a combo of both

2 tablespoons virgin coconut oil or other healthy cooking oil

½ teaspoon vanilla extract or almond extract

1 large pinch of fine sea salt

*Oats are gluten-free by nature, but most are held in facilities that contain gluten. Check the package label if you are concerned with any gluten content.

Preheat the oven to 300°F.

Combine all the ingredients in a mixing bowl. Use your clean hands to mix well and toss to coat; it will be sticky and messy, but that's the fun part. The coconut oil might be solid depending on your climate (it has a melting point of about 75°F). Your hands will warm it up and melt it into the mixture if it's solid; just be sure to mix it all through the other ingredients so there aren't any chunks of oil left.

Spread the mixture in a thin layer on a baking sheet lined with parchment paper and bake for 10 minutes, until very lightly toasted. (To make this recipe completely raw-friendly, dehydrate the mixture for 5 to 6 hours at 115°F in a food dehydrator instead.)

Cool before serving or storing. This granola can be kept in an airtight container in a cool, dry place for up to 2 weeks. I keep mine in a mason jar in the refrigerator at home and in a BPA-free plastic bag when traveling.

NOTE: Homemade granola will taste like burned popcorn if you overcook it; keep it at a low temperature for 8 to 10 minutes to let it come together.

SWEET POTATO WAFFLES

This is one of those recipes that after testing a few times, even I was surprised at how amazing the waffles turned out. Who knew the humble sweet potato could be turned into such an incredible yet healthy breakfast swap? I throw a few whole sweet potatoes in the oven if roasting veggies on Thursday or Friday to make these on Sunday morning in a snap. These waffles easily go from the freezer to the toaster to your plate.

MAKES 5 TO 6 WAFFLES

Gluten-Free, Dairy-Free, Vegetarian

WET INGREDIENTS

1 medium whole sweet potato, roasted, skin removed (about 2 cups if chopped into 1-inch pieces)

1 tablespoon virgin coconut oil

2 tablespoons real maple syrup

⅓ cup unsweetened almond milk

1 tablespoon vanilla extract

2 eggs

DRY INGREDIENTS

1 ½ cups almond flour

1 teaspoon baking soda

½ teaspoon cinnamon

¼ teaspoon salt

Roast the sweet potato whole at 400°F for 35 to 45 minutes, until you can pierce it easily with a fork. Let it cool at least 1 hour before using. It can be roasted up to 3 days in advance and stored in the refrigerator if desired.

Remove the sweet potato skin after it cools. Chop the roasted sweet potato into large chunks and add to a food processor along with the coconut oil, eggs, milk, maple syrup, vanilla extract, and cinnamon. Blend until smooth. Add the remaining dry ingredients to mixture in the food processor and blend until incorporated.

Spoon ½-cup batter into a waffle maker and cook according to the appliance's instructions, approximately 5 minutes. (I have to set my ceramic waffle maker just shy of the maximum temperature to make these waffles.) When cooked, remove the waffles from your waffle maker and place them on a cooling rack to prevent the bottoms from getting soggy from steam. Serve with real maple syrup and top with fresh berries.

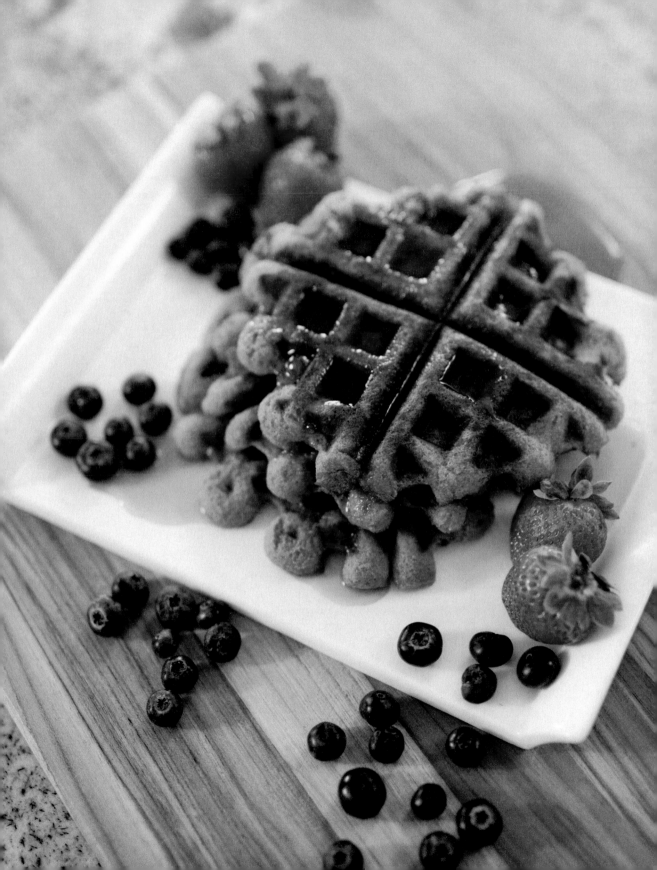

REIMAGINED HASHBROWN CASSEROLE

Hashbrown casserole is a mainstay in the American Midwest; it's known for being delicious, but also unhealthy. It gets a total revamp and healthy makeover in this new and improved recipe, which is gluten-free, dairy-free, and big on flavor. This crowd-pleaser makes an excellent breakfast or brunch, and keeps in the refrigerator all week for a simple yet hearty meal any time of day.

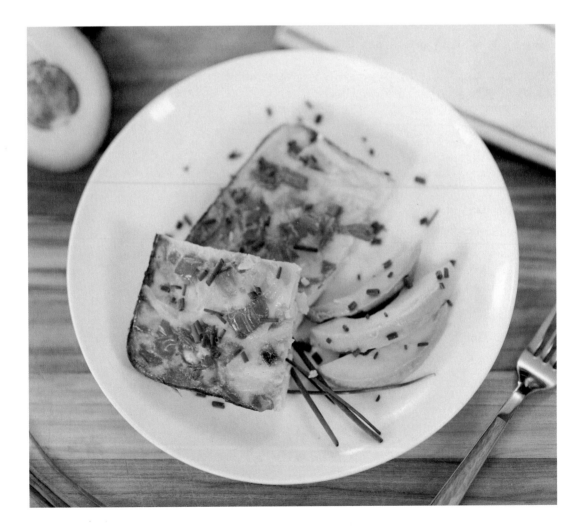

MAKES 8 TO 12 SERVINGS

Gluten-Free, Dairy-Free

VEGGIES

2 tablespoons extra-virgin olive oil (dairy-free option) or ghee (not dairy-free)

1 medium onion, chopped

1 red bell pepper, chopped

2 garlic cloves, grated or pressed

½ teaspoon sea salt

Freshly ground black pepper

CASSEROLE

One 16-ounce package organic hash browns

10 eggs, preferably organic

⅓ cup unsweetened almond milk or nondairy milk of choice

½ teaspoon sea salt

Freshly ground black pepper

Healthy cooking spray for the pan (I use grapeseed oil or extra virgin olive oil)

FOR SERVING

Chives, optional

Avocado, optional

Fermented salsa, optional

Heat 2 tablespoons oil or ghee in a sauté pan over medium heat. Add the onion, red bell pepper, and garlic and sauté 5 to 6 minutes until soft and fragrant. Turn heat to medium-low and add the garlic. Cook another 2 to 3 minutes until the garlic is fragrant. Remove from heat and allow to cool for 5 minutes (as hot veggies might pre-cook the eggs).

While the veggies cool, spread the entire package of hash browns in the bottom of a 9 x 13-inch pan sprayed with grapeseed oil or another healthy cooking spray. Layer in the (slightly cooled) sautéed veggies.

Combine the eggs, almond milk, salt, and pepper in a separate bowl. Whisk together, then pour over the hash browns and veggies. Cover and let sit overnight in the refrigerator.

The next morning, preheat the oven to 350°F. Pull the casserole dish out of the fridge to let it come to room temperature while the oven preheats. Bake for 45 to 50 minutes, until the eggs are set and the top is crisp.

Garnish with chopped chives and serve with sliced avocado and fermented salsa (or salsa of your choice), if desired.

FLEXIBLE VEGGIE FRITTATA

Mastering the art of the veggie frittata is key to every healthy cook's repertoire. Frittatas are great warm, room temperature, or cold, and they store and pack well for simple meals on the go. This no-sugar-added, balanced meal will help keep your blood sugar stable and your energy levels high. The ingredients list includes my favorite combo of veggies, but this dish is flexible, so feel free to get creative or use up leftover veggies you have on hand.

MAKES 6 SERVINGS

Gluten-Free, Dairy-Free

6 eggs

⅓ cup unsweetened almond milk

¼ teaspoon sea salt

1 tablespoon extra virgin olive oil

1 cup shredded purple sweet potato

1 cup chopped broccoli florets

4 to 5 cremini mushrooms, sliced

2 red or Swiss chard leaves, stemmed and chopped

Garlic scape, optional

About ½ teaspoon sea salt, divided

Preheat the oven to 375°F.

Preheat the oil in a sauté pan over medium heat. Sauté the vegetables with a pinch of sea salt 4 to 5 minutes or until soft.

While veggies are cooking, grate the sweet potato onto a plate or cutting board. Whisk the eggs, almond milk, and ¼ teaspoon sea salt in a medium bowl. Mix the sautéed vegetables (broccoli, mushrooms, chard, and the garlic scape, if using) with the potato and add to a 10-inch pie pan or cooked quiche crust (see recipe page 187).

Pour the egg mixture over the veggie-potato mixture. Cook for 15 to 20 minutes, until the eggs are set.

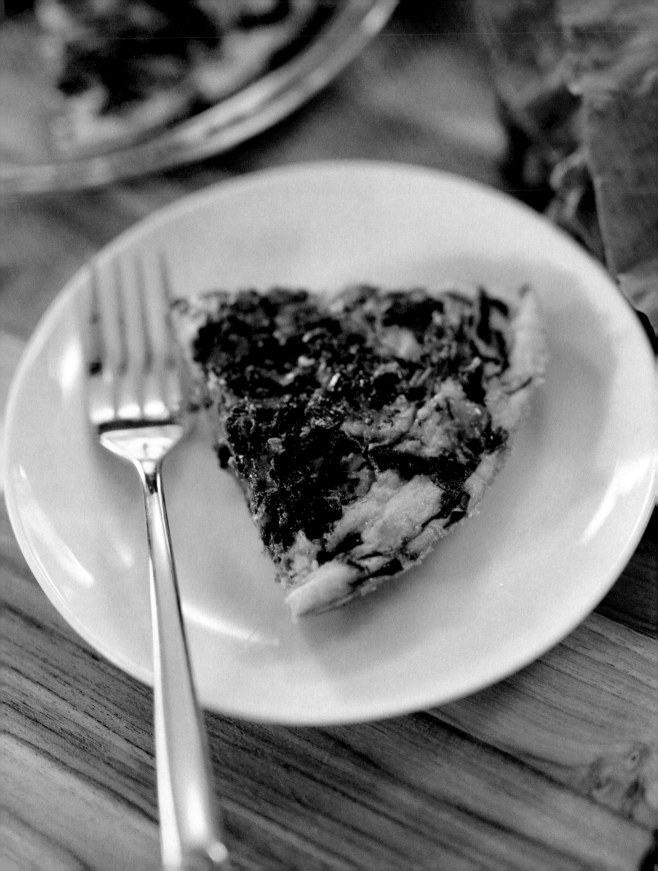

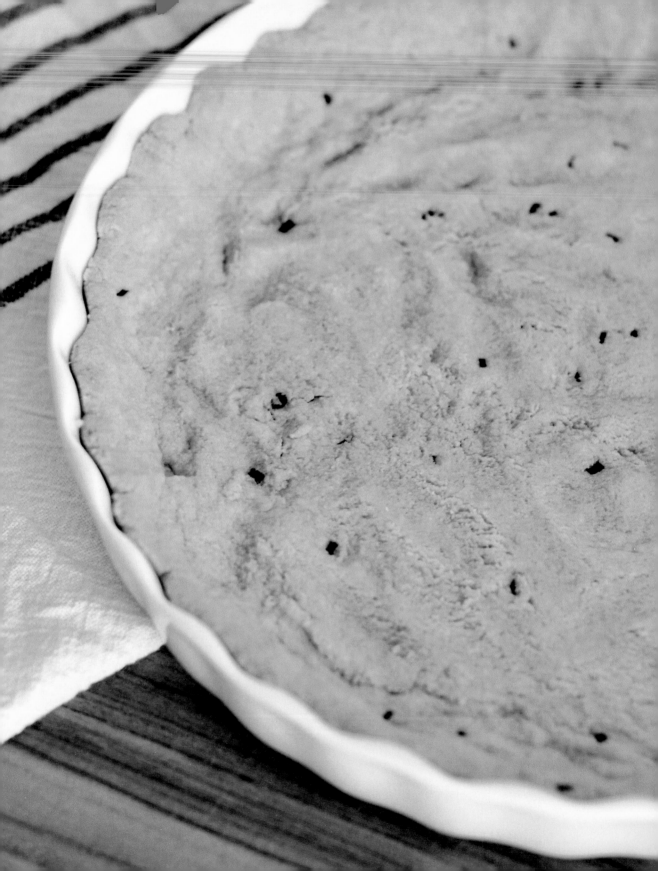

GLUTEN-FREE, DAIRY-FREE QUICHE CRUST

Turn any frittata into a healthy version of a traditional quiche by baking it inside this crust. Traditional quiche crust is made with highly processed white flour that has no nutritional benefits. Replacing it with this almond flour-based crust keeps it low-glycemic and adds nutrients, a little healthy fat, and fiber to your dish. This recipe makes one 10-inch quiche crust. It's best if left in the pan you bake it in. You can make it up to one day ahead of time, then cover and store in the refrigerator until it's time to use. This quiche crust needs to be baked before you pour the raw egg frittata mixture inside. Simply bake the crust and let it cool, then use the Flexible Veggie Frittata recipe on the previous page for the filling. This is a great way to use up any leftover sautéed or roasted veggies!

MAKES 1 10-INCH CRUST

Gluten-Free, Dairy-Free, Vegan

2 cups almond flour

½ teaspoon sea salt

½ teaspoon baking soda

¼ cup extra-virgin olive oil

2 tablespoons filtered water

1 tablespoon freshly chopped chives, optional, for an extra-savory flavor

Preheat the oven to 350°F.

Gently mix the almond flour, sea salt, and baking soda in a large mixing bowl until combined, being careful not to overpack the flour. Gently make a well in the middle of the bowl, then add the olive oil and water. Mix the ingredients with a large wooden spoon or spoon-shaped spatula until a well-combined dough forms. Transfer the mixture to a 10-inch pie pan. Using your fingers, press and shape the dough mixture about ⅛ inch thick around the pie pan and up the edges to form the crust. Bake for 12 to 15 minutes, until cooked through and set.

Let the crust cool before adding a filling such as the mixture for the Flexible Veggie Frittata (see page 184). In general, most fillings will bake for 20 to 30 minutes in a pre-cooked quiche crust. Bake until the eggs are set.

HOMEMADE COCONUT YOGURT

If you love yogurt, you're going to love this vegan option made from coconut milk. Loaded with probiotics, protein, and fiber, this recipe is sure to become a household favorite. Pair with your favorite fruits or vegetables, or use as dipping sauce for a tasty nutrient-packed snack.

MAKES 4 ½–CUP SERVINGS

Gluten-Free

2 cans coconut milk, separated (see note below)

2 grams probiotic powder*

*Make sure to use probiotic powder that contains lactobacillus bacteria.

Flip the cans of coconut milk over from how they were stored—usually the coconut water and coconut cream will separate with the cream on top. Open the cans and pour off the coconut water. Reserve the coconut water for a smoothie or other recipe.

Combine the coconut cream and probiotic powder in a clean pint-size mason jar. Place in the oven—with the oven temperature turned off, but the oven light on—for 24 to 36 hours. The probiotics will ferment the coconut cream and turn it into yogurt in the slightly warmed oven. Again, the oven should remain off, but the oven light should be on.

After 24 to 36 hours, remove the yogurt from oven and let sit 10 minutes at room temperature to cool. Taste for tanginess, which indicates that it fermented properly. It will be a little thin and runny because it is warm but will set and thicken as it cools.

Refrigerate the yogurt after it comes to room temperature (about 1 hour after you remove it from the oven). Let chill in the refrigerator at least 2 hours before serving to allow the yogurt to thicken. It will keep for 1 to 2 weeks in the refrigerator.

NOTE: For the coconut cream, use just the cream from a can of coconut milk. Refrigerate the can overnight to ensure separation of the cream from the milk.

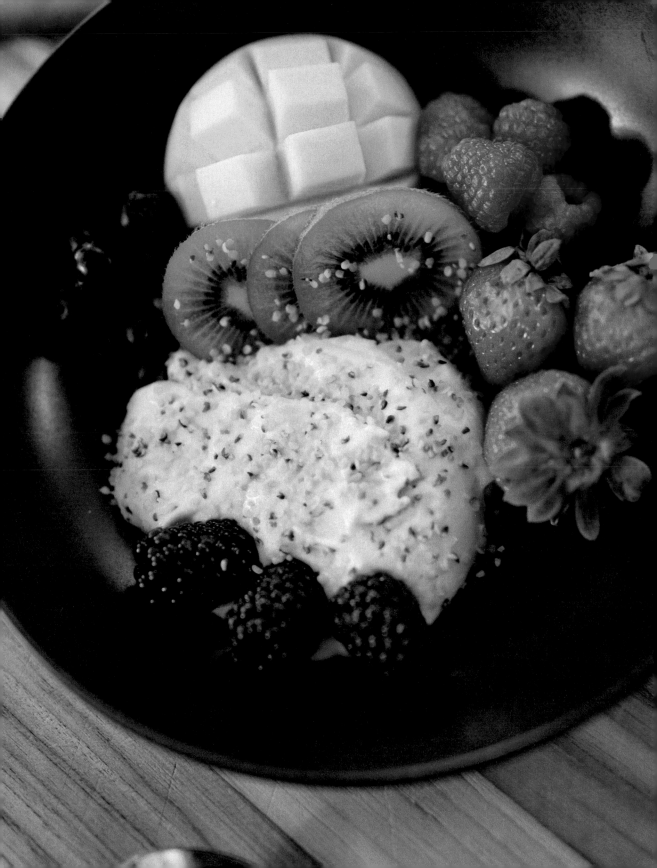

ALMOND FLOUR BREAD

If you've been looking to cut down on highly processed breads and starches, then you will love this bread. I wrote this recipe a few years ago and it's now one of the most popular almond flour bread recipes on the Internet. This version is delicious, gluten-free, and high in protein.

**MAKES 10 TO 12 SERVINGS
(1 TO 2 SLICES PER SERVING)**

Gluten-Free, Dairy-Free

2 ¼ cups blanched almond flour

¼ cup ground flaxseed

½ teaspoon baking soda

½ teaspoon finely ground sea salt (such as Real Salt)

5 eggs

½ tablespoon honey

1 tablespoon extra-virgin olive oil

1 tablespoon apple cider vinegar

Preheat the oven to 350°F. Combine the dry ingredients in a food processor and pulse them until well combined, about 10 pulses. Add the wet ingredients and mix until well combined, about 30 seconds. Scrape down the edges.

Pour the dough (it will be like a very thick batter) into a greased 9 x 5-inch bread pan; there will be enough to fill the pan about halfway up. Bake for 30 to 35 minutes, or until a toothpick inserted into the center comes out clean. Let the bread cool in the pan for 30 minutes before serving.

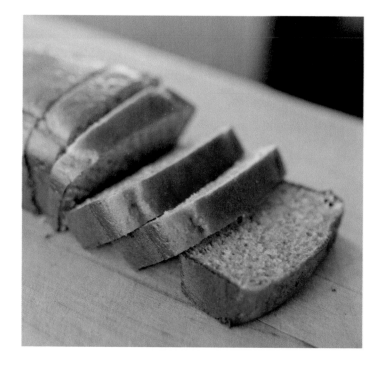

STOVE-TOP CHIA SEED JAM

Chia seed jam seems too good to be true, but it's real! I've read recipes for it over the years and I can't believe it took me this long to try it. It's seriously so easy to make and it's so good for you. I like it slathered on a fresh slice of almond flour bread.

MAKES ABOUT 10 OUNCES

Gluten-Free, Dairy-Free

2 cups frozen mixed berries

1 teaspoon fresh lemon juice

2 tablespoons raw honey, more or less to taste

2 tablespoons chia seeds

Place the fruit, lemon juice, and honey in a small saucepan over medium-high heat. Simmer for 15 minutes until the mixture bubbles and breaks down. Remove from the heat and stir in the chia seeds until well combined. Let the mixture sit for at least 15 minutes to allow the chia seeds to gelatinize.

The jam will keep in an airtight glass container in the refrigerator for up to 10 days.

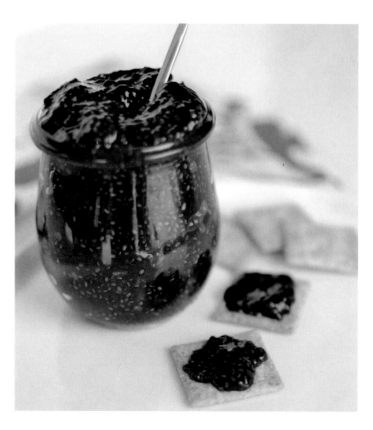

MAGIC SAUCE

I call this Magic Sauce because it tastes good on anything and everything. Use it as a dip, spread or drizzle it over roasted meat or fish. Toss roasted veggies or potatoes in it, or mix it with spaghetti squash noodles, rice noodles, or any other noodle you can think of. It's the one sauce that does it all. It also freezes well, so make a double batch for an easy meal later on. I make this year-round, and it's in heavy rotation in the spring and summer when I can grab some of the fresh herbs out of my own garden. I gently cook the garlic to infuse the oil and prevent the overpowering taste of raw garlic that you can stay with you for days. Magic Sauce instantly turns just about anything into a wow dish.

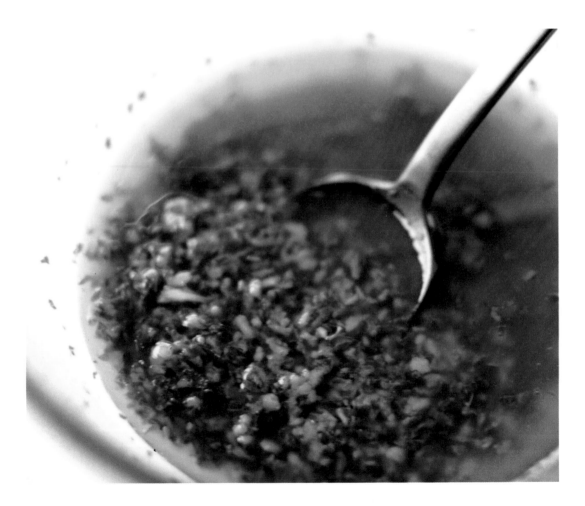

MAKES ABOUT 1 CUP (8 SERVINGS) AND CAN BE DOUBLED OR TRIPLED EASILY

Gluten-Free, Dairy-Free, Vegan

⅔ cup extra-virgin olive oil

2 garlic cloves, smashed open

¼ cup fresh basil

2 tablespoons fresh mint

1 tablespoon fresh cilantro

1 tablespoon unsalted sunflower seeds

2 inches of the white part of a scallion (green onion), chopped

½ teaspoon lemon zest

1 tablespoon fresh lemon juice

1 tablespoon red wine vinegar

½ teaspoon raw honey

Pinch of red pepper flakes

¾ teaspoon sea salt

¼ teaspoon freshly ground black pepper

Gently heat the oil in a small pan with the garlic cloves to infuse the oil with flavor and gently cook the garlic (it should not brown). Do not boil or overheat the oil. Remove from the heat and let cool while you prepare the other ingredients. Place all the remaining ingredients and the cooled cooked garlic in a food processor and pulse 8 to 10 times until well chopped. Scrape down the sides, then turn the food processor on and drizzle in the oil. Mix until saucy. You can also do this in a blender, just be careful not to over-puree—it's nice with a little bit of texture left. Use immediately or store in an airtight glass container in the refrigerator for up to 5 days. The sauce also freezes well.

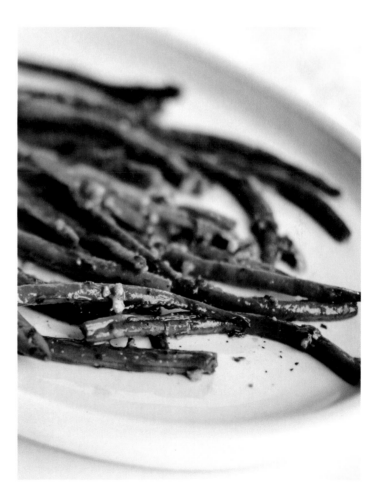

BASIC CASHEW CREAM

This is a great option for those who are looking for a vegan and dairy-free alternative to cream cheese. This easy-to-make cashew cream is a nourishing and delicious recipe that can be used as a base for other plant-based recipes.

MAKES 2 ½ CUPS

Gluten-Free, Dairy-Free, Vegan

2 cups cashews, soaked overnight or quick-soaked in hot water for 30 to 45 minutes

1 cup filtered water, more or less to blend

¼ teaspoon sea salt

Drain and rinse the cashews. Blend all the ingredients in a high-speed blender (I use a Vitamix) to a very smooth, creamy consistency. Refrigerate for up to 1 week, or freeze for up to 3 months.

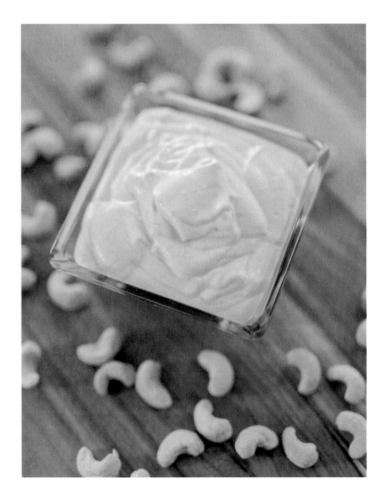

CASHEW BASIL MINT PESTO

This makes a wonderful sauce that adds a great cheesy, nutty flavor to a variety of dishes. It will quickly become a permanent addition to your family's recipe rotation.

MAKES 2 SERVINGS

Gluten-Free, Dairy-Free, Vegan

1 large garlic clove

½ cup raw cashews

¼ cup raw pumpkin seeds

2 cups fresh basil leaves

1 teaspoon lemon zest

1 lemon, juiced

¼ teaspoon sea salt, or more to taste

1 to 2 teaspoons plus ¼ cup extra virgin olive oil

Place the garlic in a food processor and run until it is well minced. Add the cashews, pumpkin seeds, basil, lemon zest, lemon juice, and sea salt. Run the food processor continuously and slowly stream in the extra virgin olive oil through the top spout. Stop and scrape down the sides.

Continue to process until the mixture is smooth, adding a touch more olive oil as needed. You may also add up to ¼ cup of water to thin down the pesto if you will be using it as a sauce.

SERVING SUGGESTION: Gently toss with spaghetti squash noodles or brown rice noodles for a delightful vegan pesto pasta.

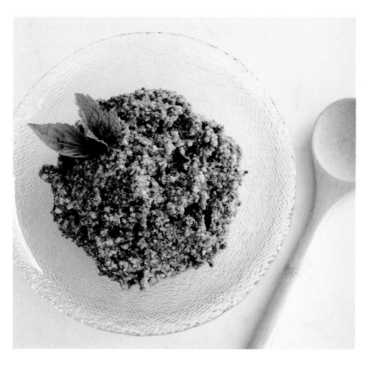

BAKED SWEET POTATO FRIES

These really hit the spot when a fry craving hits. I like to leave the skins on for extra fiber and texture. Look for long-shape sweet potatoes that are evenly round if possible, as these will give you an even cut in your fries. The key is to cut all the fries into as close to the same size as possible for even cooking, and don't put them too close together on the baking rack to prevent them from steaming.

MAKES 4 SERVINGS (THIS RECIPE CAN BE DOUBLED OR TRIPLED EASILY)

Gluten-Free, Dairy-Free, Vegan

2 medium sweet potatoes

1 ½ teaspoons extra-virgin olive oil

Sea salt

Preheat the oven to 400°F. If you have a cooling rack (the wire rack that sometimes comes with a baking sheet that you can cool cookies on), use it for even more evenly cooked fries. Line your baking sheet with parchment paper for easy cleanup. If using it, place the cooling rack over the parchment paper.

Carefully slice each cleaned and fully dried sweet potato into ¼-inch disks the long way vertically. Remove the end piece and use that as the bottom to now stack those disks and slice again the long way, leaving you with ¼-inch "fries." Toss with a small amount of extra-virgin olive oil to coat. The potatoes should be coated but not drenched as too much oil will prevent them from getting slightly crispy. Season with a few big pinches of sea salt. Arrange the potatoes on the baking rack (or directly on the parchment paper) and cook for 20 to 30 minutes, turning each fry over once halfway through. Use a set of tongs to quickly turn each one—trust me, it's worth the set for evenly cooked fries. Cook until the fries are just golden and let them cool before serving.

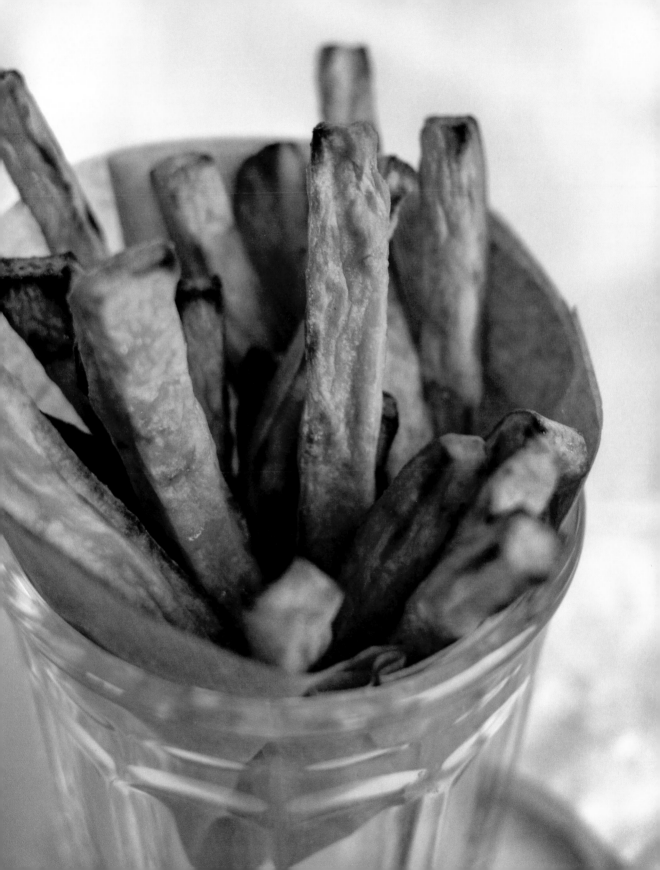

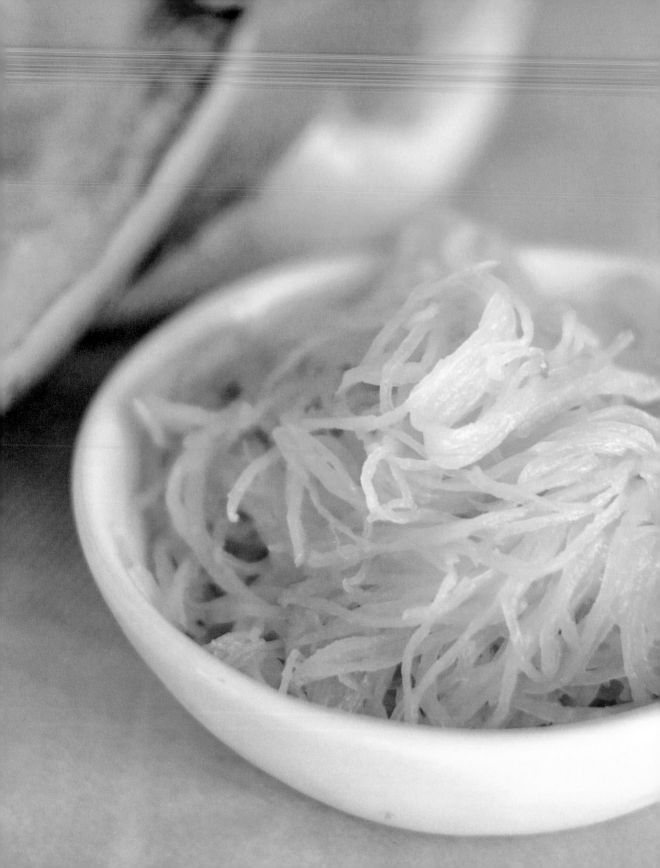

SPAGHETTI SQUASH "NOODLES"

Noodles that aren't noodles? Simply amazing. I love spaghetti squash because it has great flavor, and when it's prepared correctly, it really does have the texture of noodles. (Win.) It's also loaded with vitamins, minerals, antioxidants, and fiber. (Double win.) I like to serve this with my Cashew Basil Mint Pesto or marinara sauce.

MAKES 8 SERVINGS

Gluten-Free, Dairy-Free, Vegan

1 spaghetti squash

1 teaspoon extra-virgin olive oil

Sea salt and pepper to taste, optional

Preheat the oven to 400°F. If desired, line a baking sheet with parchment paper for easy cleanup.

Slice the top and bottom inch off the spaghetti squash. Some people prefer to leave the top on, but at least slice off the bottom to make it stable when you cut it lengthwise. Next, slice the squash in half lengthwise. Use the largest knife you have and go slow; it might take a few minutes.

Scrape out all the seeds and stringy flesh using a spoon. Brush the cut flesh of the spaghetti squash with a little extra-virgin olive oil and place it cut side down on the parchment-lined baking sheet. In very dry climates, you can add 1 or more tablespoons to the baking sheet if needed to retain moisture. I typically don't do this because I find it can make the noodles too wet, but in a very dry climate, this might help if your noodles seem too dry.

Roast the squash for 30 to 40 minutes, until the flesh is fork tender and completely cooked through. Let it rest for at least 15 minutes, or until it's cool enough to handle. Using a fork, start at one end and scrape the "noodles" out lengthwise. Voilá! You've got "noodles."

Toss with any sauce, or just a dash of extra-virgin olive oil and salt and pepper to taste. Serve hot, warm, or even chilled. Store in an airtight glass container in the refrigerator for up to 2 days.

SOCCA
(AKA CHICKPEA FLATBREAD)

If you're like I was and not familiar with socca, it's basically a hybrid between a chickpea flour pancake and flatbread. It's originally from the south of France and north of Italy (where it's called *farinata*) and served warm with herbs and often paired with a glass of rosé wine. On the health side, socca makes a fantastic naturally gluten-free flatbread, pizza crust, or bread-like snack. This recipe is written specifically for a 12-inch cast-iron skillet, which is critical to the success of this method.

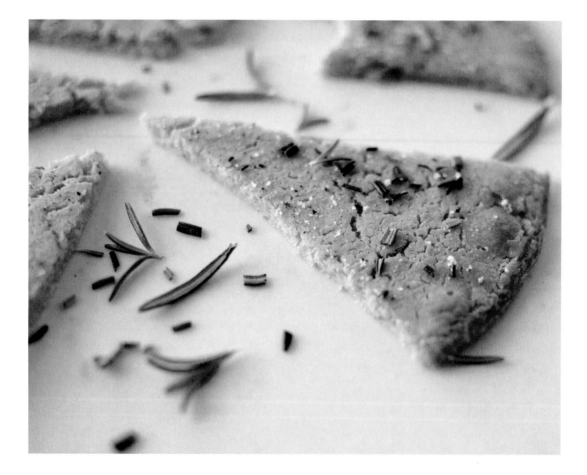

MAKES 4 SERVINGS

Gluten-Free, Dairy-Free, Vegan

1 cup chickpea flour (aka garbanzo bean flour)

1 cup filtered water, room temperature

3 tablespoons extra-virgin olive oil, divided

½ teaspoon fine sea salt (I use Real Salt)

2 tablespoons chopped rosemary or other herbs of choice for garnish

Preheat the oven to 425°F. Allow it to come up to temperature before heating your 12-inch cast iron skillet in the oven (see below).

Prepare the socca batter: Combine the chickpea flour and salt in a medium mixing bowl. Using a whisk, stir in the water until a smooth batter forms. Using the whisk, stir in 2 tablespoons extra-virgin olive oil until the batter is well combined and smooth. You don't need to whip air into the batter, the whisk just helps make it smooth.

Allow the batter to rest at least 30 minutes and up to 2 hours. This is an important step, so don't skip it; 30 minutes is just enough time to allow your oven to come up to temperature and preheat the cast-iron skillet.

Place your empty cast-iron skillet in the preheated oven (after the oven reaches 425°F) and let it heat in the oven for 15 minutes. This gets the skillet nice and hot and allows for even cooking.

Carefully remove the heated skillet from the oven with oven mitts. Swirl 1 tablespoon of extra-virgin olive oil around the hot skillet, then pour in your batter. Return the skillet to the oven and turn the oven to broil. Bake under the broiler for 7 to 10 minutes until the socca is cooked through and set. The socca is done once it pulls away slightly from the sides of the skillet and the edges are brown.

Once the socca is prepared, add your favorite toppings. I like to sprinkle mine with freshly chopped rosemary and an additional small sprinkle of sea salt.

PERFECT HOMEMADE BALSAMIC DRESSING

MAKES 1 CUP

Gluten-Free, Dairy-Free, Vegan

½ cup balsamic vinegar

½ cup extra-virgin olive oil

1 teaspoon

whole-grain mustard

¼ teaspoon sea salt

⅛ teaspoon freshly ground black pepper

Place all the ingredients in a container with a tight-fitting lid (a mason jar works great). Shake vigorously for 30 seconds until emulsified. You can also emulsify your vinaigrette in a blender or food processor (work on low, increasing the speed as you stream in the oil last). I only use a blender when working in extra-large quantities. Up to about a cup, shaking it like crazy in a mason jar works great (and there's way less cleanup).

Alternatively, you can whisk all the ingredients except the olive oil in a small bowl, then stream in the olive oil while you continue to whisk until the dressing has emulsified.

For a single serving, use 1 tablespoon each of vinegar and oil, a small dab of mustard (about ⅛ teaspoon), and just a small pinch of salt and pepper.

HEALTHY HONEY MUSTARD DRESSING

MAKES 1 CUP

Gluten-Free, Dairy-Free

¼ cup raw honey

¼ cup Dijon mustard (I prefer Sir Kensington's)

¼ cup apple cider vinegar

¼ cup extra-virgin olive oil

1 pinch of fine sea salt

A few turns of freshly ground black pepper

Whisk all the ingredients together. Alternatively, combine all the ingredients in a mason jar and shake until emulsified. Store in an airtight glass container in the refrigerator for up to 5 days.

SELF-CARE SALAD DRESSING

Want to give your body a little extra love? Try this anti-inflammatory, super-nutritious salad dressing. Not only is it packed with good-for-you ingredients, it's absolutely delicious, too. I like it tossed with a big handful of mixed baby greens (chopped) plus a big handful of arugula (chopped). I mix a tablespoon or two with the greens, and top it with a quarter of an avocado (sliced) and a few tablespoons of chopped raw nuts or seeds. It's the ultimate nourishing salad that you'll start to crave every day.

MAKES 1 CUP

Gluten-Free, Dairy-Free, Vegan

½ cup extra-virgin olive oil

¼ cup raw apple cider vinegar

1 tablespoon freshly squeezed lemon juice

¼ teaspoon freshly grated garlic

¼ teaspoon freshly grated ginger

¼ teaspoon turmeric powder

¼ teaspoon whole-grain Dijon mustard (optional and recommended)

¼ teaspoon sea salt

⅛ teaspoon freshly ground black pepper

Place all the ingredients in a container with a tight-fitting lid (a mason jar works great). Shake vigorously for 30 seconds until emulsified. You can also emulsify your vinaigrette in a blender or food processor (work on low, increasing the speed as you stream in the oil last). I only use a blender when working in extra-large quantities. Up to about a cup, shaking it like crazy in a mason jar works great (and there's way less cleanup).

Alternatively, you can whisk all the ingredients except the olive oil in a small bowl, then stream in the olive oil while you continue to whisk until the dressing has emulsified. This dressing keeps in the refrigerator in an airtight glass container for up to a week.

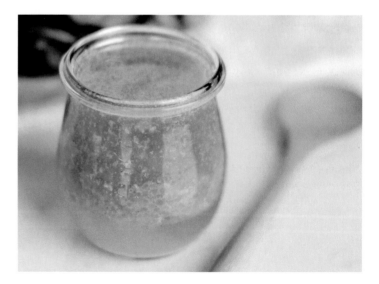

BETTER-THAN-A-BOTTLE HOMEMADE RANCH DRESSING

Once you try homemade ranch dressing, you'll never go back to the stuff in the plastic squeeze bottle again. Not only does the homemade version taste better, but it's also free of the preservatives and plastic chemicals found in the commercial stuff. Enjoy it as a salad dressing, dip, or spread.

MAKES 1 ½ CUPS

Gluten-Free, Dairy-Free, Vegan

1 cup vegan mayonnaise

1 tablespoon raw apple cider vinegar

1 tablespoon unsweetened plain nut milk or water

1 small garlic clove, finely minced or pressed, or ¾ teaspoon granulated garlic powder

1 teaspoon onion powder

2 teaspoons dried parsley

2 teaspoons fresh chopped dill

2 teaspoons fresh chopped chives

¼ teaspoon sea salt

Dash of fresh ground black pepper, to taste

Whisk all the ingredients together then transfer to an airtight glass container to store in the refrigerator—a mason jar works perfectly. Add more or less unsweetened plain nut milk or water to reach your desired consistency.

Let the dressing sit for at least 30 minutes for the flavors to develop—it's even better the next day. It will keep for about a week in the refrigerator, so halve or double the recipe as needed.

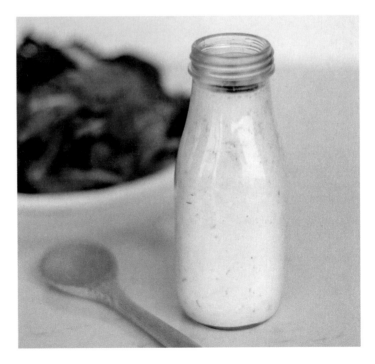

MANGO, AVOCADO & CUCUMBER SALAD

The flavors and textures in this salad are perfectly balanced, which is pretty exciting because it's as good for you as it is delicious. I love it as a snack, or a fresh summer side dish.

MAKES 5 CUPS

Gluten-Free, Dairy-Free

DRESSING

3 tablespoons fresh lime juice

3 tablespoons extra-virgin olive oil

1 tablespoon honey

¼ teaspoon fine sea salt

SALAD

1 ripe mango, peeled and chopped (about 1 ½ cups chopped)

1 avocado, chopped

1 large cucumber, halved, peeled, seeded, and chopped (about 2 ½ cups chopped)

3 tablespoons chopped cilantro

1 tablespoon chopped mint

FOR THE DRESSING: Whisk all the ingredients together in a large bowl until emulsified. (Tip: Use the same tablespoon for all measurements—if you pour the honey in the tablespoon after you've used it for the oil, it will slide out perfectly instead of sticking to the spoon.)

FOR THE SALAD: Chop all the ingredients, transfer to the bowl with the dressing, and toss gently. Store in an airtight glass container in the refrigerator for up to 3 days.

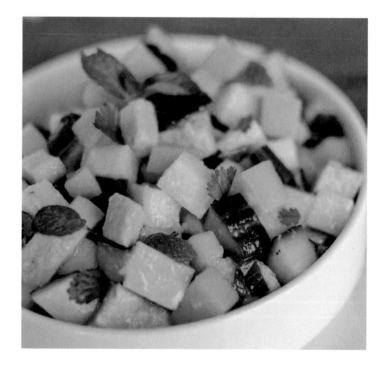

BLACK BEAN & QUINOA SALAD

This easy, delicious, and healthy dish will quickly become a new family favorite. Use it as a side dish for just about anything, or serve it up as the main event. This recipe will also show you how to make perfectly cooked, great-tasting quinoa every time. It's a great pasta replacement for gluten-conscious eaters.

MAKES 4 SERVINGS

Gluten-Free, Dairy-Free, Vegan

2 cups cooked quinoa

¼ cup extra-virgin olive oil

1 garlic clove, pressed, grated, or finely chopped

1 lime, juiced

1 teaspoon ground cumin

1 teaspoon fine sea salt

¼ teaspoon cayenne pepper, optional

Two 15-ounce cans black beans, rinsed and drained well

1 red bell pepper, chopped

6 green onions, root removed, white and part of the greens chopped

1 handful of cilantro, roughly chopped

To prepare the quinoa, rinse it well in a fine mesh colander and let all the water drain. Place the rinsed quinoa in a pot and add filtered water or vegetable stock. The ratio of liquid to quinoa is 2:1, but for the perfect fluffy quinoa, add just a tad less water. (For example, 1 cup dry quinoa needs 2 cups minus 2 tablespoons of liquid.) Bring the pot to a boil, then cover, reduce the heat to low, and simmer for about 12 to 15 minutes, or until all the liquid is absorbed and the little "tail" of the quinoa has sprouted out.

While the quinoa is cooking, whisk the olive oil, garlic, lime, cumin, and salt in a large bowl. Add the cayenne, if using. Rinse and drain the black beans, then chop the veggies.

Once the quinoa is done cooking, fluff with a fork. Add the cooked quinoa, beans, and veggies to the bowl with the dressing and gently fold it all together. Let the salad chill in the refrigerator for at least 30 minutes for the flavors to come together.

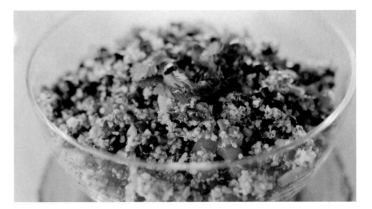

BLACK BEAN & SWEET POTATO SUPERFOOD SALAD

I've been drooling over this salad for the past two weeks, and I don't intend to stop anytime soon! Every ingredient in this dish is not only delicious, but also supports digestive and overall health. It's loaded with healthy complex carbohydrates that are naturally balanced with protein, healthy fats, and fiber to give you the fuel you need to get through the day.

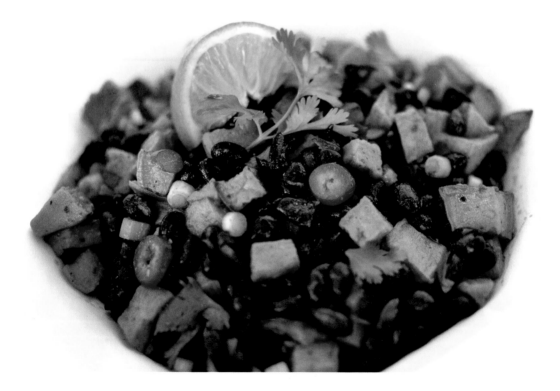

MAKES 8 SERVINGS

Gluten-Free, Dairy-Free, Vegan

1 sweet potato (either a garnet yam or white sweet potato), about ¾ to 1 pound in weight

1 ½ tablespoons extra-virgin olive oil, plus a little more for drizzling

¼ teaspoon fine sea salt, plus more to taste

A few turns of freshly ground black pepper

1 ½ tablespoons fresh lime juice (from about 1 lime)

¼ teaspoon ground cumin

¼ teaspoon ground chili powder (your choice of mild, medium, or hot)

1 garlic clove, smashed open but left whole

4 green onions, roots removed, white and green parts finely chopped (about 3 tablespoons total)

1 mild red Fresno chili pepper*

¼ cup cilantro, roughly chopped

One 15-ounce can black beans, drained and rinsed

Preheat the oven to 375°F.

Peel and chop the sweet potato into ½-inch cubes. Try to get all the pieces the same size so they roast evenly. Toss the chopped sweet potatoes with a drizzle (about 1 teaspoon) of extra-virgin olive oil, a sprinkle of sea salt, and a few turns of black pepper and place on a parchment-lined baking sheet. Spread the pieces out so they roast and don't steam. Roast for 40 minutes, or until the potatoes are soft and very slightly caramelized.

While the sweet potatoes roast, combine 1 ½ tablespoons extra-virgin olive oil, lime juice, cumin, chili powder, ¼ teaspoon sea salt, and more pepper to taste in a large bowl. Whisk to combine. Add the smashed open garlic clove and allow it to marinate in the dressing while the potatoes roast. Discard the smashed clove before combining the salad. This will infuse the dressing with garlic without overpowering the salad. For an extra-strong garlic taste, finely chop the garlic and do not remove it before tossing.

While the sweet potatoes finish roasting and the dressing marinates, chop the green onions and Fresno pepper. Roughly chop the cilantro. Drain and rinse the black beans. Reserve the ingredients in the refrigerator if not combining the salad within 20 minutes.

When the sweet potatoes are done, discard the garlic clove and add the hot sweet potatoes and black beans to the dressing first so they can soak in all the flavor. Gently toss with a large spoon. Add the chopped green onions, Fresno chili, and cilantro, and gently toss to combine.

The salad is ready to serve immediately, but I like it best if it sits in the refrigerator for at least 30 minutes for the flavors to combine. Serve as is, or over a big handful of mixed greens for a bigger meal. Store in an airtight glass container in the refrigerator for up to 4 days.

NOTES: Fresno chilis are a milder cousin of jalapeños. If you can't find a Fresno, substitute a jalapeño or a few tablespoons of finely chopped red pepper. If you're avoiding peppers or nightshades, omit the Fresno chili and chili powder altogether. Add grilled or shredded chicken breast for more protein, if desired.

CURRY QUINOA SALAD

I get a lot of requests from blog readers asking how to jazz up quinoa, and this recipe really gets the job done. It actually gets better the longer it sits; I always love it on day two. Make a big batch, and you'll have something delicious and healthy to eat all week. I adapted this recipe from Ina Garten's famous couscous salad.

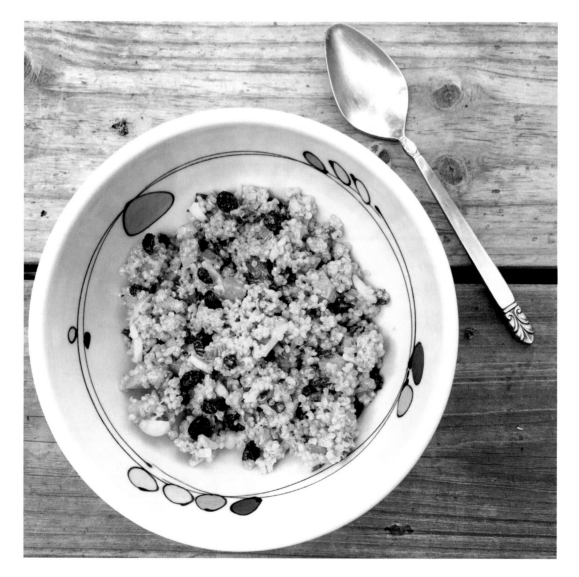

MAKES 8 SERVINGS

Gluten-Free, option for Dairy-Free and Vegan

SALAD

¾ cup dried quinoa, rinsed well

½ teaspoon sea salt

½ teaspoon mild yellow curry powder

1 ¼ cups filtered water

DRESSING

¼ cup plain unsweetened Greek yogurt*

¼ cup extra-virgin olive oil

1 teaspoon apple cider vinegar

¾ teaspoon mild yellow curry powder

¼ teaspoon turmeric

½ teaspoon sea salt

¼ teaspoon freshly ground black pepper

VEGGIES & NUTS

½ cup diced carrots (from about 2 small or 1 large carrot)

¼ cup thinly sliced scallions, white and green parts

⅓ cup dried currants or raisins

⅓ cup slivered almonds or roasted cashews

2 tablespoons chopped cilantro

*Use nondairy yogurt if you want to make this recipe dairy-free and vegan.

Place the quinoa in a fine mesh strainer or colander and rinse well until the water runs clear, about 30 seconds. Drain. Place the rinsed quinoa, salt, curry powder, and water in a medium saucepan. Bring it to a boil, then cover and reduce to a simmer. Set a timer for 12 minutes. Check the quinoa at 11 minutes—it will be done once all the water is absorbed. Be careful not to let it go too long and burn to the pan. Once all the water is absorbed, turn the heat off and fluff the quinoa with a fork. (Note: ¾ cup dried quinoa will yield 1 ½ cups cooked.)

While the quinoa cooks, whisk all the dressing ingredients in the bottom of a large mixing bowl big enough to hold the entire salad, then prepare the veggies. I find making the dressing and prepping the veggies is about the perfect amount of time to let the quinoa cook.

Once the quinoa is cooked, add it to the dressing while it's hot, then add the veggies and fold it all together. Let the salad sit for at least 30 minutes in the refrigerator to cool. This dish will keep in an airtight glass container in the refrigerator for up to 4 days.

NOTE: If you already have 1 ½ cups of prepared quinoa, just add the extra ½ teaspoon of salt and curry powder to the dressing. This salad is delicious if you can prepare the quinoa from scratch and flavor it as it cooks, but it will come together super quick and easy if you already have quinoa prepared.

EASY THAI PEANUT SLAW

This slaw is a stunner. It's also simple to make. The eye-catching colors will impress the party, and the explosion of flavors will make it a memorable dish. It's loaded with fiber and antioxidants, making it a guilt-free favorite that you can eat as often as you'd like.

The recipe will feed an army! Make it for your next gathering or as a simple make-ahead meal for your weekly meal plan.

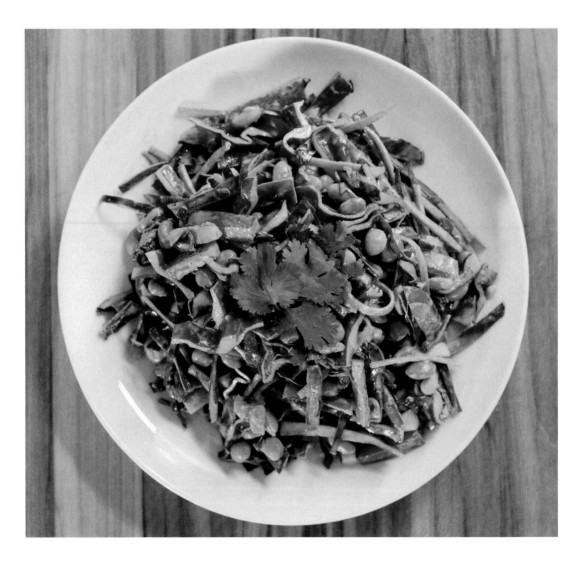

MAKES 4 SERVINGS

Gluten-Free, Dairy-Free, Vegan option

SLAW

One 10-ounce bag frozen, shelled organic edamame

4 cups shredded cabbage (any variety you like)

2 carrots, peeled and julienned or shredded (about 1 cup)

1 red bell pepper, thinly sliced (about ½ cup)

6 to 8 scallions (aka green onions), root end and 2 inches of green top removed, finely chopped

½ cup peas (fresh or frozen, defrosted in room-temperature water)

¼ to ½ cup roughly chopped fresh cilantro, to taste

SAUCE

2 tablespoons extra-virgin olive oil

2 tablespoons organic tamari (wheat-free soy sauce)

2 tablespoons raw apple cider vinegar

2 tablespoons raw honey (not vegan), maple syrup (vegan), or sweetener of choice

1 teaspoon toasted sesame oil

¼ cup creamy organic peanut (or almond) butter

1 garlic clove, peeled

1-inch piece of fresh ginger, peeled and roughly chopped

Hot sauce or a small fresh jalapeño for heat, optional

FOR THE SLAW: Soak frozen edamame in hot water to defrost. Set aside while you prepare the rest of your salad ingredients.

Wash and prepare all the produce. You can shred by hand with a sharp knife or mandoline slicer (always use the guard with a mandoline slicer to protect your hand), or use the shredding blade in a food processor.

FOR THE SAUCE: Put all the sauce ingredients in a high-speed blender and blend until smooth, about 30 seconds.

Add all slaw ingredients to a large mixing bowl. Pour the sauce on top and toss well to combine.

NOTE: The cabbage may give off water the longer it's stored. It will keep in the refrigerator for up to 3 days, and you can drain off any water as necessary.

EASY LENTIL SOUP

Lentil soup is a nutritional powerhouse. It also feeds a crowd on a tight budget. This soup combines the nutrients, protein, good carbs, and fiber in lentils with the antioxidant power of veggies, herbs, and spices. Adding a little good fat from the extra-virgin olive oil rounds it out into a perfectly balanced meal.

MAKES 8 SERVINGS

Gluten-free, dairy-free, vegan option

1 ½ cups lentils, soaked and rinsed

3 tablespoons extra-virgin olive oil

1 small yellow onion, finely chopped

2 celery ribs, finely chopped

1 large carrot, finely chopped or grated

3 to 4 garlic cloves, finely chopped

1 teaspoon ground cumin

½ teaspoon dried oregano

1 teaspoon sea salt, divided

½ teaspoon coarse black pepper, divided

1 bay leaf

1 quart vegetable stock (vegan) or chicken stock (not vegan)

2 cups filtered water

Spread the lentils out on a large sheet tray and pick out any debris (i.e., anything that doesn't look like a lentil). Legumes are harvested and stored in large quantities, and sometimes little rocks or other things make their way into the bag.

Presoaking really depends on personal preference; it helps to soften the lentils faster but is not always necessary. I typically do not presoak my lentils. If you want to soak them, pour the lentils into a large bowl and cover with filtered water so that they're submerged with an extra 2 inches on top. If you've thought ahead enough, cover the bowl with a kitchen towel and leave it on the counter for 8 to 12 hours. Drain the lentils and rinse them well before using.

While the lentils soak, heat the olive oil over medium heat in a large soup pot. Add the chopped onion, celery, and carrot and cook until tender, about 5 minutes. Add the garlic, cumin, oregano, and a pinch of both salt and black pepper to the pot. Stir and let cook for another 3 to 5 minutes, until the mixture is well combined and very fragrant. Be careful not to burn the garlic—turn the heat down if necessary, as garlic burns easily.

Add the bay leaf, the rest of the salt and pepper, the stock, water, and the soaked, rinsed lentils to the pot and bring to a full boil, then reduce the heat to a simmer. The amount of salt you need will depend on what type of stock you use—start with 1 teaspoon and add more to taste if desired.

Add the tomatoes, if using, and let the soup simmer for about 40 to 50 minutes, until the lentils are soft. Turn off the heat and stir in the vinegar.

2 tomatoes, seeded and chopped, or one 12-ounce can organic diced tomatoes, optional

1 tablespoon red wine vinegar (aged balsamic also works)

Any greens you'd like to add, optional (see note below)

Discard the bay leaf before pureeing and serving. Be very careful when blending hot mixtures, and never fill the blender/food processor more than ¼ of the way full, as hot liquids expand when blending. Depending on how you like the texture, use a handheld immersion blender to blend ⅓ to ½ of the soup. Or skip the blending if you like a firmer soup texture. If you don't have an immersion blender, puree 2 cups of the soup in a regular blender or food processor; include some of the soup's broth to blend smoothly.

If waiting longer than 1 hour to serve, leave the soup pot on the stove, but turn the burner to the lowest setting. You can leave it on the stove for 2 to 4 hours. If it gets too thick, just add another 1 to 2 cups water.

NOTE: If desired, add one handful per person of chopped greens—like spinach or kale—to the piping-hot soup a few minutes before serving for even more flavor, nutrients, and fiber. Add the greens last—once you've turned off the heat—so you don't kill all their nutrients. The greens will wilt from the heat of the soup in just a few minutes.

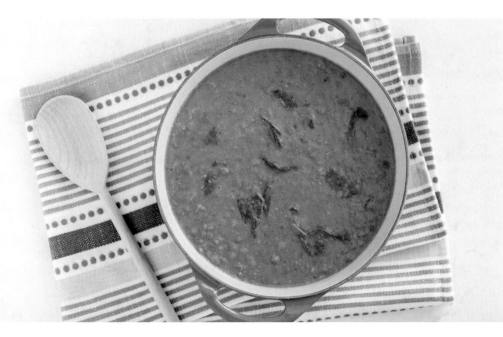

VEGAN SPLIT PEA SOUP

This soup is the perfect meal on a chilly day; it's healthy, warm, hearty, and delicious. I used to think that all the flavor in split pea soup came from the ham, but once I made it vegan, I didn't even miss the meat. I think you'll be pleasantly surprised, too.

MAKES 4 TO 6 SERVINGS

Gluten-Free, Dairy-Free, Vegan

2 tablespoons olive oil

1 medium white or yellow onion, finely chopped

1 tablespoon sea salt (more or less to taste), divided

1 medium carrot, peeled and shredded

3 garlic cloves, pressed or finely chopped

4 cups (1 quart) vegetable stock

2 cups filtered water

2 teaspoons granulated onion

1 bay leaf (fresh or dried)

2 cups dried split peas, sorted, rinsed, and soaked for 2 hours

2 teaspoons freshly ground black pepper

Heat the olive oil over medium heat in a large soup pot. Add the chopped onion and 1 teaspoon sea salt and sauté until translucent, about 5 minutes. Add the carrot and garlic and sauté another few minutes, until very fragrant.

Add the stock, water, granulated onion, remaining 2 teaspoons sea salt, pepper, and bay leaf to the pot and bring to a boil. Add the rinsed and soaked split peas and reduce the heat to medium-low. Simmer for at least 2 hours, until the peas are cooked through.

Once the peas are cooked through, remove the bay leaf and use an immersion blender to blend the soup to your desired consistency. I blend about half and leave the other half whole for a chunky texture. For a smoother texture, let the soup simmer for 4 to 5 hours and then blend until smooth.

NOTE: This soup will keep in the refrigerator for up to 3 days in a sealed glass container, or up to 3 months in the freezer.

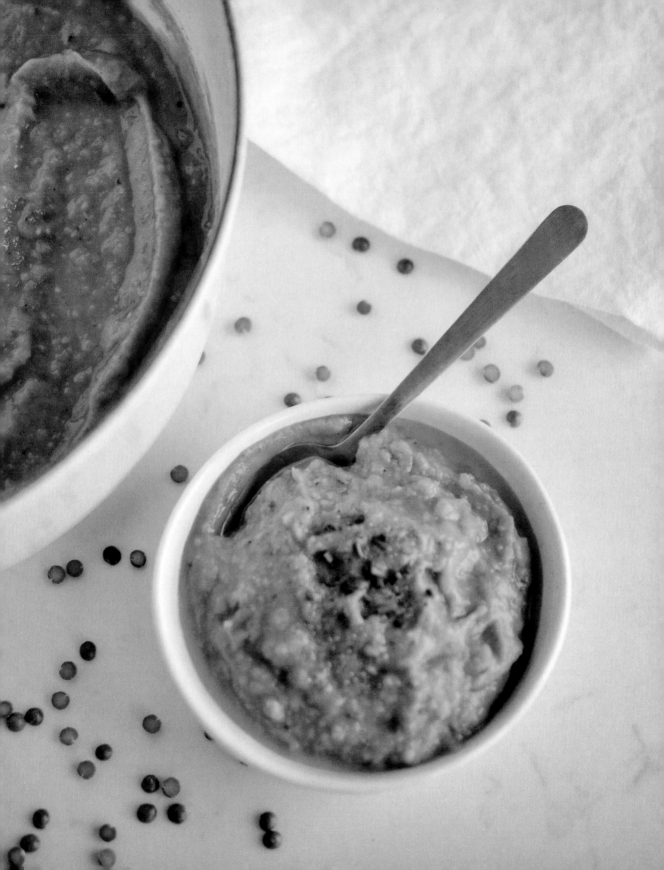

CREAMY CAULIFLOWER & LEEK SOUP

If you're craving warm comfort food that's delicious but still healthy, then this one's for you. This soup tastes a lot like baked potato soup, but instead of being high-glycemic and loaded with dairy like most creamy soups, it's actually low-glycemic and totally dairy-free!

MAKES 8 SERVINGS

Gluten-Free, Dairy-Free, Vegan option

3 tablespoons extra-virgin olive oil

1 large head of cauliflower, cleaned, green stem and leaves removed, and cut into 2-inch florets

2 large leeks (root and tough dark green tops removed), medium-chopped and cleaned

2 celery stalks, cleaned and medium-chopped

1 tablespoon fine sea salt (more or less to taste), divided

3 garlic cloves, finely chopped

1 quart vegetable stock (vegan) or low-sodium chicken stock (not vegan)

3 cups filtered water or more stock, more or less as needed

Heat the olive oil over medium-high heat in a large soup pot or Dutch oven.

To prepare the cauliflower, cut away the leaves and green part of the cauliflower stem, but use the white part of the stem—it's just as good as the florets.

To prepare the leeks, first chop, then clean them. Leeks tend to have a lot of dirt inside, so this is one veggie that you first chop, then clean. Be sure to rinse them well so you don't end up with dirt at the bottom of your soup.

Once prepared, add the leeks and celery, plus a big pinch of salt, and sauté until soft, about 5 to 6 minutes. Add the garlic, stir, and cook another minute until very fragrant, being careful not to burn the garlic. Add the stock, 2 cups water, the remaining sea salt, ½ teaspoon pepper, and bay leaf and bring to a boil. Add the cauliflower florets and reduce the heat to medium; simmer for 30 minutes, or until the cauliflower is fork-tender.

Discard the bay leaf, then puree the soup with a hand blender, or in small batches in a high-speed blender or food processor, until very smooth. A Vitamix or other high-speed blender will turn this into a very smooth soup, but a food processor or hand blender will work too, just be patient. Be very careful when pureeing hot liquid in a blender or food processor, as hot liquid expands. Never fill the blender or food processor more than ¼ full with a hot mixture. Work in very small batches until all the soup is pureed.

1 teaspoon coarse black pepper (more or less to taste), divided

1 bay leaf

1 ½ teaspoons red wine vinegar

Finely chopped chives, for garnish

Transfer the pureed soup back to the pot and stir in the vinegar and ½ to 1 cup more stock or filtered water, depending on your desired texture. Garnish with fresh chopped chives and a few dashes of hot sauce, if desired (Cholula is my favorite). The chives really make the soup amazing. Chopped parsley or raw pumpkin seeds are also great additions.

This soup can be stored in the refrigerator in an airtight glass container for up to 3 days. It also freezes well.

NOTE: You'll need about 7 to 8 cups of liquid to make this soup and you can use all stock or a combination of stock and water. If you use water, consider adding a vegetable bouillon cube to the simmering soup.

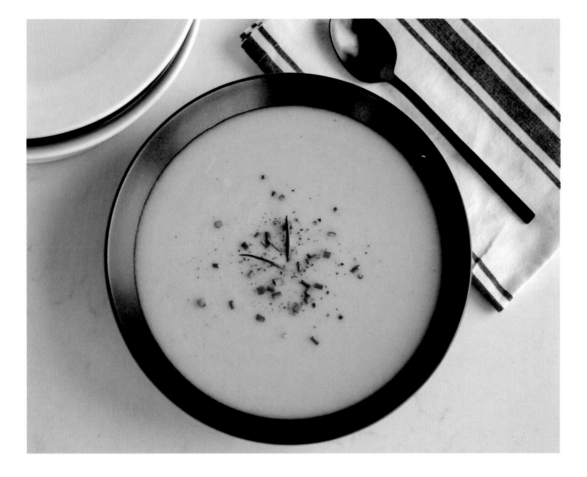

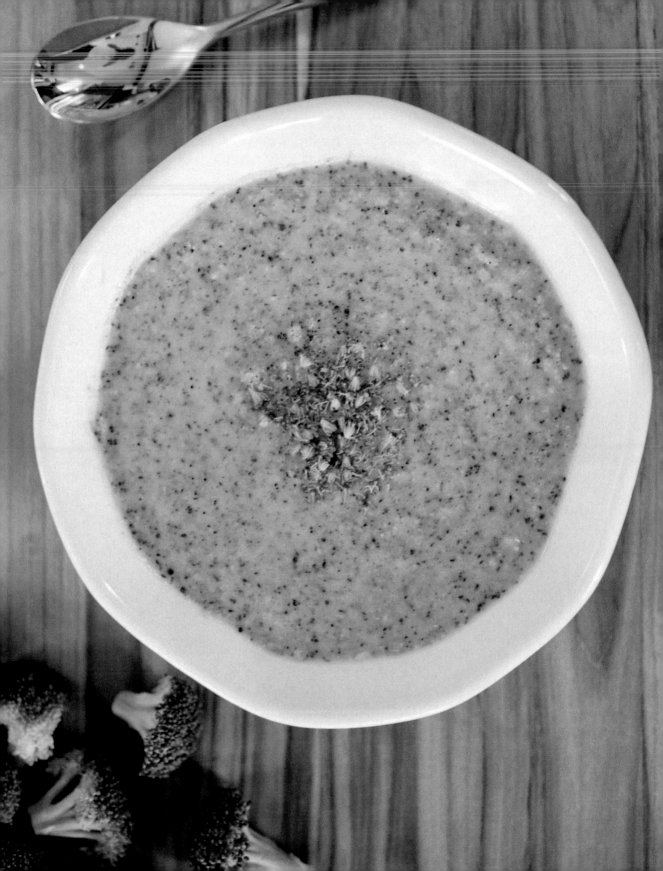

ULTIMATE BROCCOLI "CHEEZE" SOUP

Broccoli has never tasted so good! I promise you this creamy soup will be a hit with the kids, too. You don't need dairy to make soups creamy. With this recipe, you can make a hearty broccoli soup full of flavor with aromatic spices and homemade cashew cream.

MAKES 8 SERVINGS

Gluten-Free, Dairy-Free, Vegan option

SOUP

2 tablespoons extra-virgin olive oil

1 medium brown or white onion

Large pinch of sea salt, plus more to taste

1 medium carrot, grated or finely chopped

2 garlic cloves, pressed, grated, or finely chopped

3 cups broccoli florets

2 cups cauliflower florets

Freshly ground black pepper

3 cups unsalted bone broth (not vegan), chicken stock (not vegan), or vegetable stock (vegan), divided, plus 1 cup for the cashew cream below

CASHEW CREAM

½ cup cashews, soaked

1 cup bone broth (not vegan) or vegetable stock (vegan)

2 tablespoons nutritional yeast

½ teaspoon sea salt

FOR THE SOUP: Preheat the olive oil in a large Dutch oven over medium heat. Sauté the onion with a large pinch of sea salt until soft and fragrant. Add the carrots and cook until soft. Add the garlic and cook another minute. Add the broccoli, cauliflower, more sea salt to taste, and black pepper and cook for 2 to 3 more minutes. Add 3 cups broth to the mixture and bring to a simmer. Simmer for 20 to 25 minutes, until the broccoli and cauliflower florets are tender and can be pierced with a fork.

FOR THE CASHEW CREAM: Puree the cashews in a high-speed blender with 1 cup broth, nutritional yeast, and sea salt until the cashews are emulsified into a cream. Leave the cashew cream in the blender and pick out the cooked cauliflower florets (it's okay if some broccoli comes along), adding to cream. Puree until smooth.

Reserve the cream and cauliflower mixture in another bowl, then add the cooked broccoli, veggies, and broth to the blender. Pulse a few times until coarsely pureed. Add the broccoli mixture and the cream mixture back to the pot and stir together until heated through. Serve the soup hot, or store in the refrigerator for up to 5 days. It also freezes well.

NOTE: You can choose to soak your cashew nuts overnight, otherwise you can do a quick soak, where you use hot water and soak for 1 hour.

CHICKEN POBLANO CHILI

This dish is a one-pot wonder. It's filling, satisfying, and healthy. I love making this on Sunday for dinner, then storing the rest in the refrigerator for lunch on Tuesday or Wednesday (if it lasts that long).

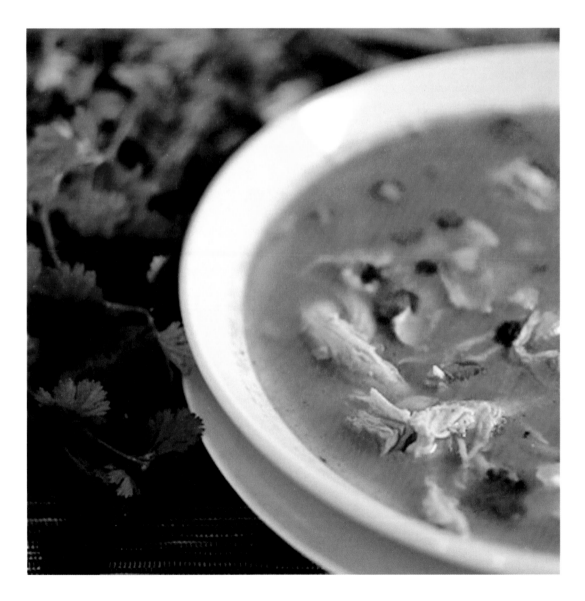

MAKES 8-PLUS SERVINGS

Gluten-Free, Dairy-Free,
Vegan option

1 large poblano pepper

2 tablespoons extra-virgin
olive oil

1 small white or yellow onion,
chopped

3 garlic cloves, pressed,
grated, or finely chopped

1 ½ teaspoons ground cumin

1 teaspoon chili powder of
your choice

Large pinch of sea salt, plus
more to taste

Small pinch of freshly ground
black pepper, plus more to
taste

1 quart organic chicken
stock (not vegan) or
vegetable stock (vegan)

2 cups filtered water

Two 15-ounce cans cannellini
beans, drained and rinsed
well

1 pound boneless skinless
chicken breasts (about 2
breasts; omit if making this
recipe vegan)

Avocado, fresh cilantro,
and fresh organic corn for
garnish, optional

Roast the poblano pepper either over the flame on your gas burner or under the broiler, turning every few minutes until it's charred all the way around, about 5 minutes total. Place the hot charred pepper in a glass bowl and cover the bowl (plastic wrap works great) to trap the steam for at least 15 minutes but up to 1 day ahead. Once steamed, peel the charred skin off and discard. Remove and discard the stem and seeds.

Heat 2 tablespoons extra-virgin olive oil in a large soup pot over medium heat. Add the onion and sauté for 3 to 4 minutes, or until soft. Reduce the heat and add the garlic, cumin, chili powder, large pinch of sea salt, and small pinch of freshly ground black pepper. Cook the garlic and spices with the onions for 2 to 3 minutes, then add the stock, water, and beans. Bring to a boil, then reduce to a low simmer.

Once at a low simmer, add the chicken breasts, if using, to the pot and poach them gently. Always poach at a low simmer to prevent the meat from becoming tough. Check at 30 minutes. Once the chicken is cooked through, remove it from the pot and shred with two forks. Set aside until after the poblano is pureed.

Place the roasted poblano in a blender with 3 large ladles full of the soup mixture (stock, beans, onions, and spices, but none of the chicken). Leave at least half of the beans in the pot to leave them whole. Puree the poblano with the beans and soup mixture to create a thick and creamy base. Add the shredded chicken and pureed mixture back into the pot and stir. Add more salt and pepper to taste. Garnish with avocado, fresh cilantro, and fresh organic corn if desired.

MOM'S HOMEMADE CHICKEN STOCK (AKA BONE BROTH)

Once you learn how to make this chicken stock, you'll be hooked for life. There's a reason that chicken stock is used as the base for so many soups and sauces; it has a delicious flavor and is wonderfully nutritious.

MAKES ABOUT 4 QUARTS

Gluten-Free, Dairy-Free

1 whole chicken (about 4 to 5 pounds), any paper inside removed

1 white or yellow onion, quartered

2 carrots, scrubbed or peeled and cut in half

2 celery stalks (with leaves if possible), cut in half

4 to 5 garlic cloves, smashed open or cut in half

1 large bay leaf

3 to 5 sprigs fresh thyme

5 stems fresh parsley (about 1 small handful)

2 teaspoons sea salt

½ teaspoon whole black peppercorns

1 tablespoon apple cider vinegar

2 lemon slices, optional

Enough filtered water to fill the pot

You'll need a 6- to 8-quart pot with a tight-fitting lid—I use a 6-quart pot for a 4- or 5-pound chicken. Be sure to check the inside of the chicken and remove the paper pouch that contains the organs. Discard the paper and the organs if desired. Alternatively, you can add the organs to the pot. If you're new to stock, this might sound strange, but there is a lot of great nutrition in there.

This recipe uses a whole chicken so that you can use the meat in soup or another recipe, but you can also use this recipe with any bones that you have, like from a leftover roasted chicken or turkey. Just use whatever is left from the whole chicken or turkey after you've removed the meat. If you don't have access to fresh herbs, you can use a large pinch of dried herbs instead. Get creative if you want! Use whatever root veggies or herbs that you have on hand or like the flavor of.

Add all ingredients to the pot and cover with filtered water to about an inch below the top of the pot. Put a tight-fitting lid on the pot, set it on the stove, and bring to a boil (this takes about 10 to 20 minutes), then reduce it to a simmer. Simmer for at least 4—and up to 24—hours. If you use a whole chicken, be sure to remove the meat from the chicken about 2 hours in to prevent it from overcooking, then put the bones back in the pot to continue cooking.

To remove the meat, carefully remove the whole chicken from the pot and set it on a large cutting board. It will be very hot, so let it cool a bit so that you can handle it. Use 2 forks or a knife to remove as much meat as possible. The meat will be nicely poached, and you can shred it or just cut it up. Put the meat in an airtight glass container, then let it come to room temperature before you store it in the refrigerator where you can keep it for up to 3 days. Or, use it immediately.

Then put all the bones and skin and the whole body back into the pot and let it simmer for at least another 2 hours. You can simmer your stock for 4 to 24 hours. The longer you simmer it, the more flavorful and nutritious it will be. Keep the pot covered to prevent your stock from evaporating; if you notice the liquid reducing too much you can add a few more cups of water at any time during the process.

After simmering the stock for at least 4 hours, strain it through a fine mesh colander or cheesecloth into a large bowl or pot. Discard everything that was in the pot except the liquid you just strained—it's all served a very useful purpose, and by now, the veggies have been boiled to the point that they will fall apart.

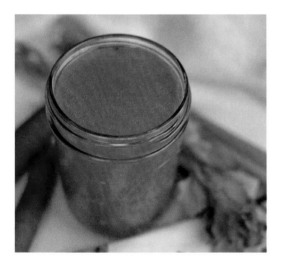

SLOW-COOKER METHOD

Follow the above directions but use a slow cooker instead.

Add all the ingredients and water to your slow cooker and put it on high until it comes to a simmer, about 2 hours. It will take a while to simmer as the slow cooker heats at a slower pace than your stove top.

Remove the meat once it's cooked through, about 2 to 3 hours in. Add everything back in just like the method above, and let it all simmer on low for 4 to 24 hours. You may want to add another cup or 2 of filtered water if you let it simmer overnight and too much liquid evaporates. Just keep it covered and let it simmer as long as you'd like. All slow cookers (aka Crock-Pots) are different—you may want to leave it on high if it's not gently simmering on low. I leave mine on low overnight after being on high for about 3 hours, and it simmers all night.

Use your stock right away to make homemade chicken soup. To store, let it come to room temperature and then transfer it to quart-size containers. It will keep in the refrigerator for up to 3 days, or in the freezer for up to 6 months. If freezing, it's best to freeze in portions that will be convenient to use in recipes, like 2-cup or 4-cup/1-quart containers.

HOMEMADE THAI RED CURRY

Move over take-out. Grab a can of organic coconut milk and prepare to be amazed: I'll show you how to make decadent (yet healthy!) homemade curry loaded with veggies and chickpeas.

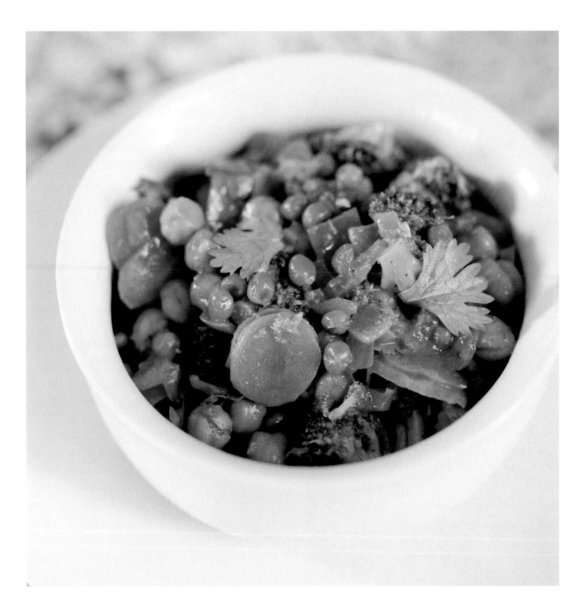

MAKES 4 SERVINGS

Gluten-Free, Dairy-Free, Vegan option

1 red bell pepper, diced

1 head of broccoli, florets cut and stalk cut into thin coins

2 large carrots, cut into thin coins

½ large onion

1 tablespoon dry red curry powder or 1 ½ tablespoons curry paste

1 cup brown rice

1 tablespoon coconut oil

2 teaspoons sea salt, more or less to taste

2 garlic cloves, or more to taste

1-inch piece of ginger, skin removed

One 14-ounce can of full-fat coconut milk

½ cup plus one tablespoon filtered water, divided

1 tablespoon raw honey (not vegan), maple syrup (vegan), or sweetener of choice

½ teaspoon turmeric powder

One 15-ounce can of chickpeas, drained and rinsed

½ cup frozen sweet peas

Fresh cilantro, for garnish

Dice the bell pepper into approximately ½-inch pieces. Cut florets from the broccoli. Remove the thick skin from the outside of the stalk with a knife or vegetable peeler, then thinly slice the stalk on an angle with a mandolin or a sharp knife. Next, peel the carrots and slice thinly on an angle with a knife or mandolin. Dice the onion into approximately ½-inch pieces.

Mix the dry curry powder and water until it forms a paste. Use a one to one ratio of powder to water to mix the paste.

Prepare the rice in a pot or a rice cooker.

Melt 1 tablespoon coconut oil in a large sauté pan over medium heat. Add the onions and a pinch of sea salt and sauté until the onions are soft and slightly translucent, about 3 minutes. Turn the heat to medium-low, then grate the garlic and ginger directly into the pan. Stir to combine and let the mixture sit for approximately 1 minute, then add the curry paste and another pinch of sea salt. Sauté for an additional 1 minute to let the spices toast.

Add 1 can of coconut milk and ½ cup water to the pan. Once the coconut milk has melted, add the honey and turmeric powder; let this mixture come to a gentle simmer. Add the chickpeas, carrots, bell pepper, and broccoli, along with another pinch of sea salt, and stir to combine. Cook for approximately 20 minutes for an al dente texture on the vegetables. Add the frozen peas and let them warm through before serving. Add more salt to taste.

Serve the curry over brown rice (or cauliflower rice or quinoa) and top with fresh cilantro.

UNFRIED CAULIFLOWER "FRIED RICE"

Craving take-out but want to stay on track? This one really hits the spot for Chinese take-out but without the crazy amounts of sugar, sodium, processed carbs, or MSG. This extra-light recipe is made with cauliflower rice, but check out my website for the brown rice version if you want another variation.

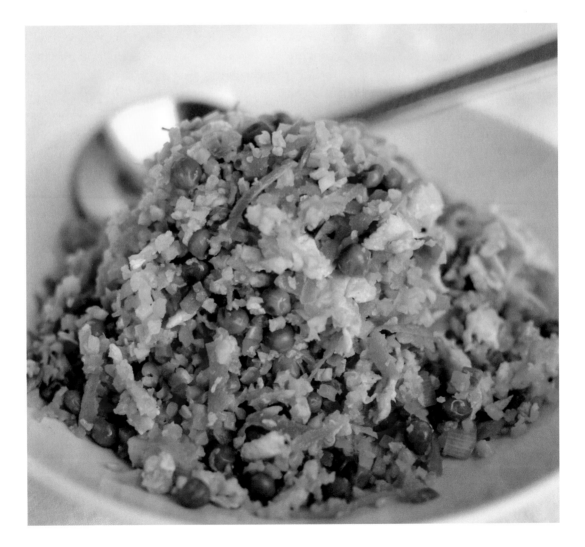

MAKES 4 SERVINGS

Gluten-Free, Dairy-Free,
Vegetarian

1 tablespoon macadamia nut
oil or avocado oil (or other
healthy cooking oil), divided

2 large eggs

Sea salt

Freshly ground black pepper

5 scallions (aka green
onions), root and 2 inches
of green tops removed,
chopped (about ½ cup)

1 large carrot, shredded or
julienned (about 1 cup)

½ cup frozen peas

½ teaspoon freshly grated
ginger

½ teaspoon freshly grated
garlic

3 tablespoons organic tamari
(see Notes) or low-sodium
soy sauce

1 teaspoon apple cider
vinegar

1 teaspoon toasted sesame
oil

3 cups cooked cauliflower
rice (fresh or frozen)

Heat ½ tablespoon oil over medium heat in a medium sided skillet.

Whisk the eggs in a mixing bowl until well combined and season to taste with a pinch each of salt and pepper. Add the eggs to the pan and scramble. Once cooked remove the scrambled eggs from the pan to a plate and reserve.

Add the remaining ½ tablespoon oil to the pan over medium heat; add the scallions and carrot and sauté 3 to 4 minutes until softened. Add the frozen peas, ginger, and garlic to the pan. Sauté 1 to 2 minutes, until fragrant. Add the tamari, apple cider vinegar, and toasted sesame oil. Stir well to combine once, then add the cauliflower rice. Cook about 5 minutes until the rice has absorbed all the liquid. Turn off the heat and stir in the scrambled eggs until well combined.

NOTES: Tamari is gluten-free soy sauce that tastes just like regular soy sauce. You can find it in the ethnic food aisle of most grocery stores or at an Asian market. You can also substitute coconut aminos for a completely soy-free version.

I've made this with both frozen cauliflower rice (found in the freezer section) and fresh cauliflower rice (often labeled "riced cauliflower," found in the fresh produce section). I prefer the texture of this dish with the fresh (not frozen) version, but frozen works well, too. You can also buy a whole head of cauliflower and grate it with a cheese grater to make your own cauliflower rice, but the packages are fresh and much easier. One 12-ounce bag of cauliflower rice is generally 3 cups.

SECRET-INGREDIENT TUNA BOATS

No time to cook? No problem. This is an easy-to-assemble dish that doesn't require any cooking. It can be made ahead of time and it's a recipe that's easy to double. The secret ingredient, fermented pickle relish, adds an extra dose of gut-healthy probiotics to this seemingly simple dish.

MAKES 3 TO 4 SERVINGS

Gluten-Free, Dairy-Free

6 to 8 romaine leaves, rinsed and dried

2 cans albacore tuna, drained

2 tablespoons finely chopped celery

3 tablespoons healthy mayonnaise (I prefer Vegenaise)

1 ½ tablespoons unsweetened fermented pickle relish

¼ to ½ teaspoon sea salt

Pinch of black pepper

1 teaspoon raw local honey

TOPPINGS

8 grape tomatoes, halved

1 avocado, diced

Rinse the romaine leaves, and spin-dry in a salad spinner or pat dry with paper towel.

Drain the liquid from the tuna cans and add the tuna to a mixing bowl. Break up the larger chunks with a fork until the tuna is evenly flaky. Add the celery, mayonnaise, fermented pickle relish (our secret ingredient!), salt, and pepper to the tuna and mix well.

To assemble, lay out your individual leaves of romaine lettuce and add a scoop of tuna to each. Top with tomatoes and avocado. Store any leftover tuna for up to 2 days in the refrigerator.

NOTE: The dressing will keep for about a week in the refrigerator, so halve or double the recipe as needed.

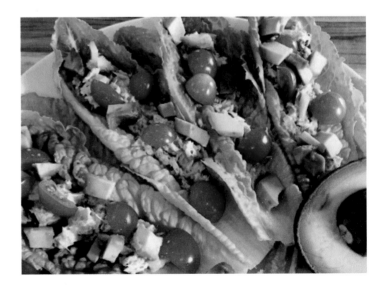

10-MINUTE MAPLE DIJON SALMON

With three simple ingredients you probably already have in your refrigerator you can make restaurant-worthy salmon in less than 20 minutes.

MAKES 2 SERVINGS

Gluten-Free, Dairy-Free

Two 6- to 8-ounce salmon fillets

Sea salt

Freshly ground black pepper

2 teaspoons real maple syrup

2 teaspoons organic tamari (wheat-free soy sauce)

2 teaspoons Dijon or whole-grain mustard

Position your oven rack approximately 6 inches below the broiler. Preheat the oven to 300°F. Once the oven is preheated, turn it off and turn the broiler on. Line a baking pan with a sheet of parchment paper (optional). Place the salmon fillets on the baking pan skin-side down. Lightly coat the fillets with sea salt and freshly ground black pepper.

Whisk the maple syrup, tamari, and mustard in a small mixing bowl for the marinade. Coat the salmon with the marinade, then place in the oven and broil for 6 minutes, or until cooked through. Let the salmon cool for 5 to 10 minutes before serving.

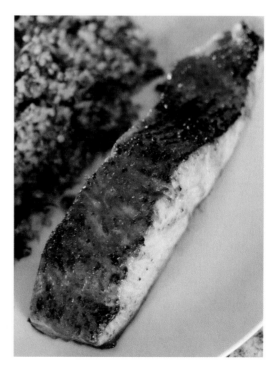

HEALTHY SLOW-COOKER CHICKEN TACOS

Insanely delicious healthy chicken tacos in less than 25 minutes of hands-on time? Count me in. This no-fuss recipe will be your new #TacoTuesday go-to for sure, and no one even has to know that you prepared it on Sunday.

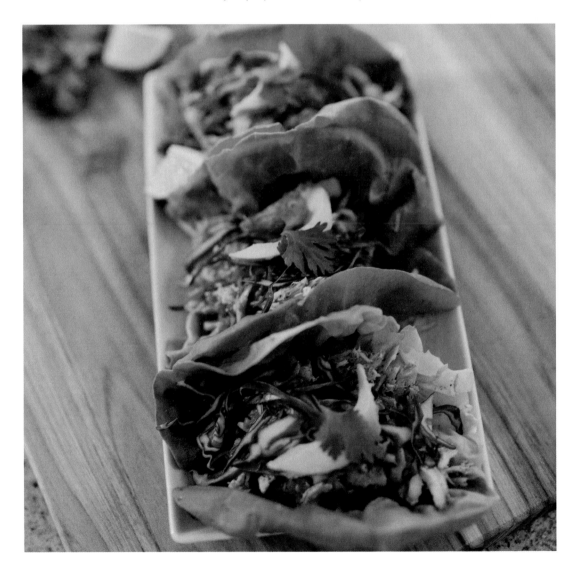

MAKES 8 SERVINGS (CAN BE SCALED UP OR DOWN EASILY)

Gluten-Free, Dairy-Free

1 cup filtered water or chicken stock

3 garlic cloves, smashed

2 tablespoons mild or medium chili powder

1 tablespoon plus 1 teaspoon ground cumin

2 teaspoons sea salt

4 to 5 turns of freshly ground black pepper

1 medium onion, cut into quarters

2 pounds boneless skinless chicken breasts, preferably organic (that's about 4 to 5 chicken breasts)

1 to 2 limes, juiced for garnish

SERVE WITH

Butter lettuce or romaine lettuce leaves, or your favorite healthy tortillas

Fermented salsa or pico de gallo

Shredded cabbage

Avocado

Cilantro

Mix the water, garlic, chili, cumin, salt, and pepper in a medium bowl. Place the chicken breasts in a slow cooker (aka Crock-Pot). Pour the liquid mixture over the chicken and top with the onion. Cook for 2 to 3 hours on high, or 4 to 5 hours on low, until the internal temperature of each breast reaches 165°F.

Shred the chicken with 2 forks. Squeeze the lime juice over the meat before serving. Serve in lettuce cups or your favorite tortillas with salsa, shredded cabbage, avocado, and cilantro.

GAME-DAY CHILI

This is my easy go-to healthy game-day chili recipe. I usually have most of the ingredients on hand, and it's a cinch to pull together. It also feeds an army, so make it for a party or as a make-ahead meal for a few nights that week.

MAKES 10 SERVINGS

Gluten-Free, Dairy-Free

1 pound organic grass-fed ground beef (85 or 90% lean), optional

Sea salt (about 2 to 3 teaspoons total for the whole pot)

Freshly ground coarse black pepper

1 yellow or white onion, chopped

1 carrot, grated or finely chopped

2 to 3 garlic cloves, pressed or grated

2 tablespoons chili powder

2 teaspoons ground cumin

1 bay leaf

2 15-ounce cans tomato sauce

2 15-ounce cans diced San Marzano tomatoes (or 4 large fresh tomatoes, diced)

1 15-ounce can black beans, drained and rinsed

1 15-ounce can kidney beans, drained and rinsed

Preheat a large Dutch oven to high heat. Brown the meat, if using, for 2 to 3 minutes until slightly caramelized. Add a healthy pinch of sea salt and a sprinkle of black pepper and stir. Reduce the heat to medium. (If you're making this chili vegan, place about 1 tablespoon olive oil in the pot then proceed to the next step.)

Add the onion and carrot. Stir and cook until soft, 3 to 4 minutes. Add the garlic, chili powder, cumin, bay leaf, cinnamon (if using), and a pinch of sea salt and stir for about 1 minute to cook the garlic and toast the spice. Reduce the heat while cooking the garlic if needed so it doesn't burn.

Bring the pot back to medium heat; add the tomato sauce and diced tomatoes (the acid from the tomatoes will deglaze the bottom of the pot). Stir well, scraping the bottom of the pot.

Add the beans and peppers, plus 1 teaspoon salt and ½ teaspoon pepper. Stir well and cook for at least 5 minutes, then taste to see if you need more salt. I usually end up adding another teaspoon of sea salt, but depending on how much you used earlier and the other ingredients, you may not need it. Don't be afraid to salt your food! Salt brings out the flavor of all foods, and cooking from scratch won't even come close to the sodium levels in processed foods. Add 1 cup of filtered water to thin out your chili if it is too thick.

Let the chili simmer on low (stirring about every 15 minutes) for at least an hour to let the flavors come together. The longer it sits, the better the flavor will be. If you make it a few hours ahead, you can turn the heat on a covered Dutch oven off for a

1 15-ounce can pinto beans, drained and rinsed

1 red bell pepper, chopped

1 jalapeño, chopped (optional, for heat)

⅛ teaspoon ground cinnamon, optional (it's delicious, I promise!)

GARNISHES

Sliced avocado

Chopped cilantro

Finely diced red onion

A few organic corn tortilla chips (I like the extra-thin ones)

few hours and it will stay hot. Just turn the heat back on a few minutes before you're ready to serve. Or, keep it in a Crock-Pot on the warm setting on your counter or transport to the tailgate. There are tons of options here.

Store any leftovers in an airtight glass container for up to 3 days in the refrigerator or up to 3 months in the freezer.

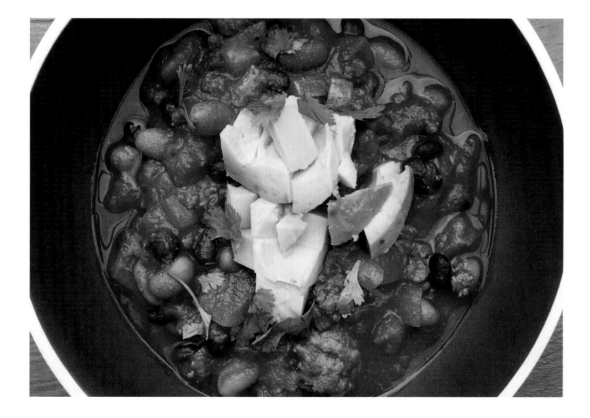

NO-BAKE EXTRA-CHOCOLATEY CHOCOLATE AVOCADO MOUSSE

This recipe proves that avocados are a miracle food. The mousse is so decadent and smooth that it's hard to believe that it's vegan, let alone good for you. A small serving is a great after-dinner treat that not only satisfies your chocolate craving, but beautifies your skin while you sleep.

MAKES 6 TO 8 SERVINGS

Gluten-Free, Dairy-Free, Grain-Free, Nut-Free, Vegan

2 ripe avocados, peeled and pitted

2 tablespoons coconut cream

1 frozen banana

⅓ cup raw cacao

⅓ cup 100 percent pure maple syrup (substitute with another frozen banana for no sugar added)

2 teaspoons high-quality vanilla extract

Big pinch of fine sea salt

Blend all the ingredients on high in a food processor or high-speed blender until smooth. Top with strawberries, or eat it as is. The mousse will keep in the refrigerator for up to 4 days, or in the freezer for up to 4 months.

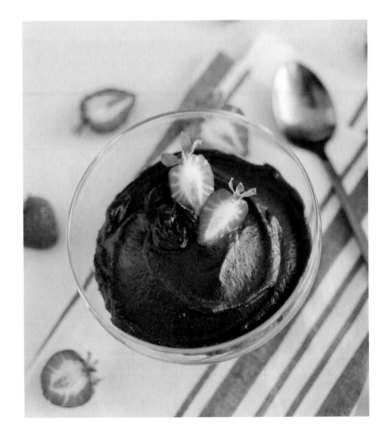

NO-BAKE KEY LIME MOUSSE

Light and fluffy, just the way a mousse should be, you'll never believe how healthy this version is!

MAKES 8 SERVINGS

Gluten-Free, Dairy-Free, Vegan option

1 cup cashews, soaked overnight or quick-soaked

2 large avocados

¼ cup raw honey (not vegan) or maple syrup (vegan)

1 teaspoon lime zest

⅓ cup lime juice

¼ teaspoon sea salt

½ cup filtered water

Ginger, optional

Blend all the ingredients in a high-speed blender until smooth. Serve immediately or refrigerate. The mousse will keep in the refrigerator for up to 24 hours and freezes well.

NOTE: You can choose to soak your cashew nuts overnight, otherwise you can do a quick soak, where you use hot water and soak for 1 hour.

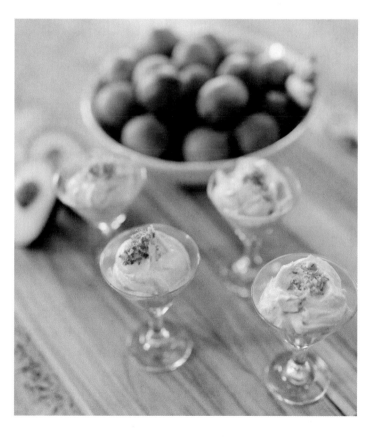

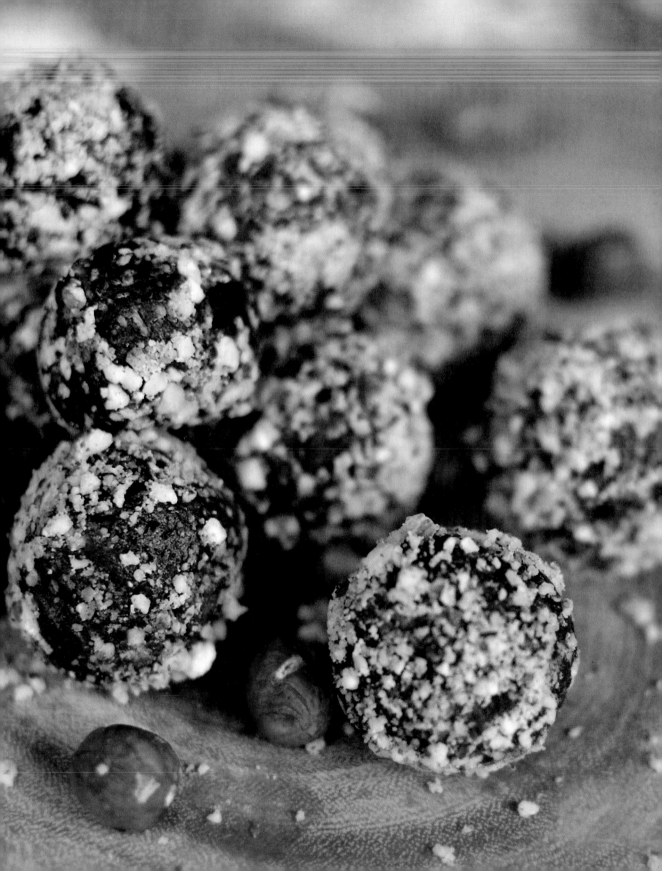

NO-BAKE CHOCOLATE HAZELNUT ENERGY BITES

Tired of boring health food snacks? Try these easy, addictive, on-the-go energy bites; they're like a party in your mouth. Using fiber- and mineral-rich dates as a base, this chocolatey snack satisfies your sweet tooth and provides extra energy for your busy lifestyle.

MAKES 24 BALLS

Gluten-Free, Dairy-Free, Vegan

¼ cup hazelnuts

15 dates, pitted

2 tablespoons cacao (raw chocolate) powder or unsweetened cocoa powder*

¼ cup unsweetened almond butter

2 tablespoons chia seeds

1 tablespoon coconut oil

½ teaspoon pure vanilla extract

Sea salt

*Make sure the cocoa does not contain any milk ingredients to make this recipe dairy-free and vegan.

Blend the hazelnuts into a medium-fine powder in a food processor. Overall, it should be an even grind. Remove the blade from the food processor and transfer the ground hazelnuts to a plate, where the energy bites will be rolled out.

Put the blade back in your food processor and the add dates, cacao, almond butter, chia seeds, coconut oil, vanilla, and salt. Run the food processor for 1 minute, then stop and scrape down the sides; this may be repeated once or twice. Once the mixture forms a ball, it should be done.

Transfer the mixture to a cutting board. Roll the mixture into balls with the palms of your hands, then roll the balls in the ground hazelnuts until evenly coated. Place all the energy bites on a baking sheet lined with parchment paper and refrigerate for 1 hour. Serve or store in a glass container in the refrigerator for up to 1 week.

DELICIOUSLY HEALTHY
APPLE CRISP

This recipe proves that healthy eating requires no sacrifice. One blog reader commented, "This recipe is amazing! I am not gluten-free but have two close friends who are, so I made this for them and tried it myself—somewhat skeptically—and it blew me away! My husband even loved it too!"

MAKES 8 SERVINGS

Gluten-Free, Dairy-Free,
Vegan options

FILLING

4 firm, tart apples (about 1 ½ pounds), such as McIntosh, Granny Smith, or Pink Lady, peeled* and sliced thin

½ teaspoon grated orange zest (optional but recommended)

1 teaspoon grated lemon zest

2 tablespoons freshly squeezed lemon juice (zest the lemon first)

2 tablespoons filtered water (or bourbon or brandy for an adult twist)

2 teaspoons arrowroot starch or 1 tablespoon gluten-free flour mix

½ teaspoon ground cinnamon

½ teaspoon ground nutmeg or pumpkin pie spice

Preheat the oven to 350°F.

Peel the apples if desired. I like to peel 2 apples and leave the skin on the other 2. Slice the apples into thin (about ⅛ inch) slices. Place the apples in a large mixing bowl. Add the rest of the ingredients for the filling and toss to coat all the apple slices. Pour the apples into an 8x8-inch (or 8-inch round) baking dish. Put the apples—uncovered—in the oven for 15 minutes while you make the topping to allow them to start releasing their juices.

For the topping, combine all the ingredients except the butter, and mix well until large crumbles form. Use your fingers or a knife to sprinkle chunks of the butter into the mixture; it should still resemble large crumbles.

Carefully remove the apples from the oven. Sprinkle the topping mixture evenly over the apples, covering the fruit completely. Place the dish back in the oven. Bake for 40 more minutes to 1 hour, until the top is golden brown and the fruit is bubbly. Check the topping 30 minutes after putting it in the oven. The topping should be crispy and lightly golden. If the topping is getting too dark or crispy, cover it with foil for the rest of the baking time. The apples will continue to release juice and soften, so bake no less than 50 minutes total for the best texture.

Serve warm with coconut whipped cream or vegan vanilla ice cream of your choice.

½ teaspoon high-quality vanilla extract, optional (use Madagascar vanilla for the best flavor)

1 big pinch of fine sea salt

½ cup real maple syrup (vegan) or honey (not vegan)

TOPPING

1 cup almond flour

1 cup whole rolled oats (use certified gluten-free oats if gluten-free is desired)

½ cup chopped pecans

⅓ cup real maple syrup (vegan) or honey (not vegan)

⅓ cup coconut crystals (aka coconut sugar)

½ teaspoon cinnamon

½ teaspoon fine sea salt

3 tablespoons cold unsalted grass-fed butter (not vegan) or vegan butter (like Earth Balance), diced, or ½ cup coconut oil (vegan)

*You can peel the apples or not. I like to peel half and leave the skin on the other half; the skin is full of fiber and adds nice texture.

NOTES: To make this recipe no-sugar-added, eliminate the maple syrup and coconut crystals. It will be different and not as sweet, but still delicious.

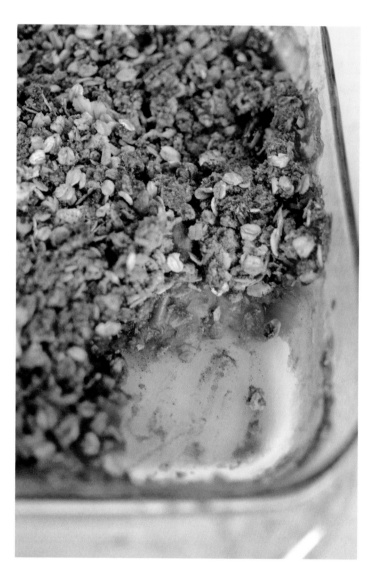

NO-BAKE VEGAN RASPBERRY CHEESECAKE

I'm in love with this healthy dessert! I'm calling it a cheesecake because it looks like one, but it doesn't contain any dairy or processed ingredients. It's a no-bake treat that's full of healthy ingredients and comes together in less than 15 minutes of hands-on time.

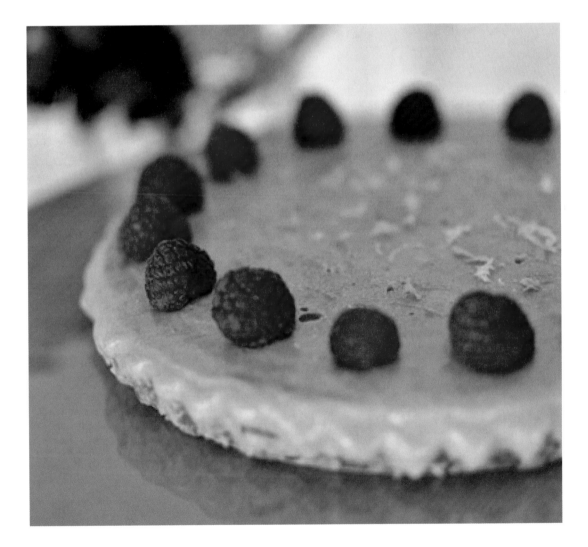

MAKES 8 SERVINGS

Gluten-Free, Dairy-Free, Vegan

CRUST

½ teaspoon virgin coconut oil to grease the pan (grapeseed oil or almond oil will work, too)

¾ cup whole raw almonds

3 Medjool dates, pitted

½ teaspoon vanilla extract

Pinch of sea salt (about ⅛ teaspoon)

FILLING

Coconut cream from 1 can of organic coconut milk*

½ cup raspberries, fresh or frozen, plus ⅓ cup fresh berries for garnish

6 Medjool dates, pitted

2 teaspoons fresh lemon juice

1 teaspoon vanilla extract

Pinch of sea salt (a scant ⅛ teaspoon)

½ teaspoon lemon zest for garnish, optional

*For the coconut cream, you'll want to use a can of full-fat coconut milk and let the coconut water separate from the cream in the can. To ensure that this happens, place the can in the refrigerator overnight. If the contents don't separate, you can use the unseparated milk, the filling just won't be as thick.

Grease a 7-inch tart pan with ½ teaspoon virgin coconut oil. An 8-inch pan will work, too; the cheesecake will just be a little thinner.

Pulse all the crust ingredients in the food processor until the almonds are very finely chopped—about 20 pulses, or 45 seconds. Be careful not to turn the mixture into almond butter; it should still have a texture to it. Press the crust into the tart pan with your fingers. Freeze for 30 minutes, or up to 24 hours, before you fill it. Cover the crust with plastic wrap if you plan to freeze it longer than an hour before filling.

Open the can of coconut milk upside down and pour the coconut water into a separate container so you can use just the cream. (Reserve the coconut water for a smoothie or another recipe.)

Place all the filling ingredients in a blender and blend until smooth, about 60 to 90 seconds. Pour the filling into the frozen crust, cover with plastic (a gallon-size plastic freezer bag works great), and freeze for at least 2 hours. Eat the cheesecake within 3 days of making it, letting the cheesecake sit at room temperature for about 10 minutes to soften slightly before serving, garnishing the edges with fresh raspberries and lemon zest, if desired. It won't melt as fast as ice cream, but the dessert will eventually melt, so store it back in the fridge or freezer as needed.

RESOURCES
& RECOMMENDATIONS

Multivitamins & Supplements:
elizabethrider.com/supplements

Savings on Healthy Groceries:
elizabethrider.com/thrivemarket

Healthy Beauty Product Choices:
elizabethrider.com/beautyfavorites

Book Recommendations:
elizabethrider.com/bookrecommendations

Become a Health Coach:
elizabethrider.com/healthcoach

Learn how to build a blog & online business:
elizabethrider.com/business

Join Elizabeth's VIP list for free at elizabethrider.com/start for more healthy recipes, wellness inspiration and subscriber-only updates.

ENDNOTES

Introduction

1. "Preventable Deaths from Heart Disease and Stroke," CDC VitalSigns, September 2013, https://www.cdc.gov/VitalSigns /pdf/2013-09-vitalsigns.pdf; and Centers for Disease Control and Prevention, "Heart Disease Facts," https:// www.cdc.gov/heartdisease/facts.htm.

2. "From high intensity exercise to 'sleep debt': Biochemist reveals the six things you do every day that are ageing you—and how to stop them," DailyMail.com, August 15, 2018, https://www.dailymail.co.uk/femail/article-6061245; and Dr. Libby Weaver, *The Beauty Guide* (Little Green Frog Publishing, 2018). https://www.drlibby.com/shop /the-beauty-guide/.

3. R. Brown, et al., "Secular differences in the association between caloric intake, macronutrient intake, and physical activity with obesity," *Obesity Research & Clinical Practice* 10, no. 3 (May–June 2016): 343–255. https://www .sciencedirect.com/science/article/pii/S1871403X15001210.

Chapter 2

1. World Health Organization, "Guideline: Sugars Intake for Adults and Children," 2015, https://www.who.int /nutrition/publications/guidelines/sugars_intake/en/.

2. S. Mihrshahi et al., "Fruit and vegetable consumption and prevalence and incidence of depressive symptoms in mid-age women: Results from the Australian longitudinal study on women's health," *European Journal of Clinical Nutrition* 69, no. 5 (May 2015): 585–91. https://www.ncbi .nlm.nih.gov/pubmed/25351653.

3. U.S. Food and Drug Administration, "Sodium," https://www .accessdata.fda.gov/scripts/InteractiveNutritionFactsLabel /factsheets/Sodium.pdf.

4. Harvard T.H. Chan School of Public Health, "Health Risks and Disease Related to Salt and Sodium," https://www .hsph.harvard.edu/nutritionsource/salt-and-sodium /sodium-health-risks-and-disease/.

Chapter 3

1. Statista, "Market value of packaged food in the United States from 2013 to 2018 (in million U.S. dollars),*" https://www.statista.com/statistics/491685 /packaged-food-united-states-market-value/.

2. G. Rubin, "Back by Popular Demand: Are You an Abstainer or a Moderator," Gretchen Rubin (blog) (October 10,

2012), https://gretchenrubin.com/2012/10/back-by-popular-demand-are-you-an-abstainer-or-a-moderator/.

3. H. Armitage, "Low-fat or low-carb? It's a draw, study finds," Stanford University School of Medicine, February 2018, http://med.stanford.edu/news/all-news/2018/02/low-fat-or-low-carb-its-a-draw-study-finds.html.

4. The University of Sydney, GI News: Glycemic Index, http://glycemicindex.com/.

5. C. Petersen and J. L. Round, "Defining dysbiosis and its influence on host immunity and disease," *Cellular Microbiology* 16, no. 7 (July 2014): 1024–1033. https://www.ncbi.nlm.nih.gov/pmc/articles/PMC4143175/.

Chapter 4

1. I. Janssen et al., "Waist circumference and not body mass index explains obesity-related health risk," *American Journal of Clinical Nutrition* 79, no. 3 (March 2004): 379–84. https://www.ncbi.nlm.nih.gov/pubmed/14985210.

2. M. Roth et al., "Self-Detection Remains a Key Method of Breast Cancer Detection for U.S. Women," *Journal of Women's Health* 20, no. 8 (August 2011): 1135–1139. https://www.ncbi.nlm.nih.gov/pmc/articles/PMC3153870/.

3. "Time for more vitamin D," Harvard Women's Health Watch, September 2008, https://www.health.harvard.edu/staying-healthy/time-for-more-vitamin-d.

4. American Thyroid Association, "Prevalence and Impact of Thyroid Disease," https://www.thyroid.org/media-main/press-room/.

5. S. Consul et al., "Comparative study of effectiveness of Pap smear versus visual inspection with acetic acid and visual inspection with Lugol's iodine for mass screening of premalignant and malignant lesion of cervix," *Indian Journal of Medical and Paediatric Oncology* 33, no. 3 (July–September 2012): 161–65. https://www.ncbi.nlm.nih.gov/pmc/articles/PMC3523473/.

6. American Autoimmune Related Diseases Association, "How many Americans have an autoimmune disease?" April 29, 2017, https://www.aarda.org/knowledge-base/many-americans-autoimmune-disease/.

Chapter 5

1. Environmental Working Group, "Exposures add up – Survey results," EWG's Skin Deep Cosmetics Database (June 15, 2004), https://www.ewg.org/skindeep/2004/06/15/exposures-add-up-survey-results/.

Chapter 6

1. Centers for Disease Control and Prevention, "Sleep and Sleep Disorders," https://www.cdc.gov/sleep/index.html.

2. D. Benson, "Trouble sleeping? Experts say skip antihistamines," Baylor College of Medicine, October 7, 2013, https://www.bcm.edu/news/sleep-disorders/experts-warn-against-antihistmaines-sleep-aid.

3. R. Oliveira, "What About 10,000 Steps a Day?" UC Davis Integrative Medicine, June 15, 2016, https://ucdintegrativemedicine.com/2016/06/10000-steps-day/#gs.jrPb7vc.

4. University of California - Irvine, "Even mild physical activity immediately improves memory function: Now you just need to remember to exercise!" ScienceDaily, September 24, 2018, https://www.sciencedaily.com/releases/2018/09/180924153424.htm.

5. K. Ishikawa-Takata et al., "How much exercise is required to reduce blood pressure in essential hypertensives: a dose–response study," *American Journal of Hypertension* 16, no. 8 (August 1, 2003): 629–633. https://academic.oup.com/ajh/article/16/8/629/199247.

6. American Cancer Society, "Diet and activity factors that affect risks for certain cancers: Breast cancer," https://www.cancer.org/healthy/eat-healthy-get-active/acs-guidelines-nutrition-physical-activity-cancer-prevention/diet-and-activity.html.

7. T. P. Aird, et al., "Effects of fasted vs fed-state exercise on performance and post-exercise metabolism: A systematic review and meta-analysis," *Scandinavian Journal of Medicine & Science* in Sports 28, no. 5 (May 2018): 1476–1493. https://www.ncbi.nlm.nih.gov/m/pubmed/29315892/.

Chapter 8

1. M. Grothaus, "Why Journaling Is Good for Your Health (And 8 Tips to Get Better)," Fast Company (January 29, 2015), https://www.fastcompany.com/304148%-tips-to-more-effective-journaling-for-health; N. Farber, "The Law of Attraction Revisited," *Psychology Today* (blog) (January 5, 2014), https://www.psychologytoday.com/us/blog/the-blame-game/201401/the-law-attraction-revisited.

2. AJ Adams, "Seeing Is Believing: The Power of Visualization," *Psychology Today* (blog) (December 3, 2009), https://www.psychologytoday.com/us/blog/flourish/200912/seeing-is-believing-the-power-visualization.

RECIPE INDEX

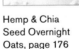

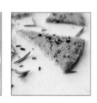

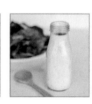

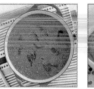

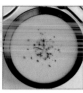

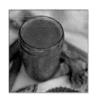

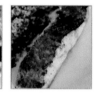
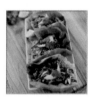

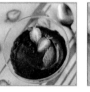

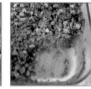

INDEX

ACKNOWLEDGMENTS

I am eternally grateful for the support I had while writing this book. My deepest gratitude goes to my mom, for endless encouragement, and teaching the value of real food and hard work, and to my dad, for always believing in me and supporting every decision I've ever made. Angela and Kara, thanks for being the best sisters a little sister could ask for, and for always celebrating my successes. Support from my family and friends gave me the confidence to create this book.

A book like this one takes a village to create. Many thanks to Samantha Lord for capturing photographs that so brilliantly tie together the words of this book; D'Arcy Benincosa for the cover; Kelsey Eads for helping with the food shots; Kate Lindsay; Elizabeth Dellwo; and Kendra Springer for assisting me to get ready for photoshoot days.

My deepest gratitude goes to Sue Ward, M.S., Director of Nutrition at Sanoviv Medical Institute for reviewing the nutrition information presented in this book.

Thanks to everyone at Hay House who helped make this book a reality. Special thanks to Mary Norris, my editor and book doula; Patty Gift for taking a chance on a first-time author without a fully formed outline; Lisa Cheng for her guidance and attention to detail; Tricia Breidenthal and Shubhani Sarkar for working with me to design a book that showcases my words on paper; and all the other editorial and production professionals for catching every last detail.

And last but not least, thank you to all of my clients, customers, blog readers, and current (and future) book readers who continue to support my work and online community. This book wouldn't exist without you. It's an honor to be your health coach.

Elizabeth Rider is a leading nutrition and whole-living expert teaching women around the world how to become the healthiest, most successful versions of themselves. In a world flooded with diet information, Elizabeth's healthy recipes and straightforward nutrition advice draw millions of inspired readers to her popular blog.

Best known for her fun and accessible approach to food and healthy living, she's built an online wellness empire from scratch on her iPhone and laptop. Thousands have had success using her online programs, which include The Health Habit Hub, Clean Up Your Diet, and The Wellness Business Bootcamp.

As host of *Elizabeth Eats* on Food Matters TV, Elizabeth is delightfully changing the way the world views healthy home cooking. She speaks on stages around the world and mentors scores of ambitious people each year to seek and live life on their own terms.

As a Certified Holistic Health Coach (Integrative Nutrition) and accomplished online entrepreneur, cultivating a lifestyle of freedom and health is her religion. Elizabeth is a graduate of Cornell University's Plant-Based Nutrition program and a TEDx speaker. Her recipes have been featured on Shape.com, The Zoe Report, Forbes, MindBodyGreen, Buzzfeed, and Greatist, among others.

Visit her at ElizabethRider.com.

HAY HOUSE TITLES OF RELATED INTEREST

———

YOU CAN HEAL YOUR LIFE,
the movie, starring Louise Hay & Friends
(available as a 1-DVD program, an expanded 2-DVD set, and an online streaming video)
Learn more at www.hayhouse.com/louise-movie

THE SHIFT, the movie,
starring Dr. Wayne W. Dyer
(available as a 1-DVD program, an expanded 2-DVD set, and an online streaming video)
Learn more at www.hayhouse.com/the-shift-movie

CRAZY SEXY JUICE:
100+ Simple Juice, Smoothie & Nut Milk Recipes to Supercharge Your Health,
by Kris Carr

THE EARTH DIET:
Your Complete Guide to Living Using Earth's Natural Ingredients,
by Liana Werner-Gray

MEDICAL MEDIUM LIFE-CHANGING FOODS:
Save Yourself and the Ones You Love
with the Hidden Healing Powers of Fruits & Vegetables,
by Anthony William

THE TAPPING SOLUTION FOR WEIGHT LOSS & BODY CONFIDENCE:
A Woman's Guide to Stressing Less, Weighing Less, and Loving More,
by Jessica Ortner

———

All of the above are available at your local bookstore or may be ordered by visiting:

Hay House USA: www.hayhouse.com®
Hay House Australia: www.hayhouse.com.au
Hay House UK: www.hayhouse.co.uk
Hay House India: www.hayhouse.co.in

We hope you enjoyed this Hay House book. If you'd like to receive our online catalog featuring additional information on Hay House books and products, or if you'd like to find out more about the

Hay Foundation, please contact:

Hay House, Inc., P.O. Box 5100, Carlsbad, CA 92018-5100
(760) 431-7695 or (800) 654-5126
(760) 431-6948 (fax) or (800) 650-5115 (fax)
www.hayhouse.com® • www.hayfoundation.org

——

Published in Australia by: Hay House Australia Pty. Ltd.,
18/36 Ralph St., Alexandria NSW 2015
Phone: 612-9669-4299 • *Fax:* 612-9669-4144
www.hayhouse.com.au

Published in the United Kingdom by: Hay House UK, Ltd.,
The Sixth Floor, Watson House, 54 Baker Street, London W1U 7BU

Phone: +44 (0)20 3927 7290 • *Fax:* +44 (0)20 3927 7291
www.hayhouse.co.uk

Published in India by: Hay House Publishers India,
Muskaan Complex, Plot No. 3, B-2, Vasant Kunj, New Delhi 110 070
Phone: 91-11-4176-1620 • *Fax:* 91-11-4176-1630
www.hayhouse.co.in

——

Access New Knowledge.

Anytime. Anywhere.

Learn and evolve at your own pace
with the world's leading experts.

www.hayhouseU.com

Free e-newsletters
from Hay House, the Ultimate
Resource for Inspiration

Be the first to know about Hay House's free downloads, special offers, giveaways, contests, and more!

 Get exclusive excerpts from our latest releases and videos from *Hay House Present Moments*.

 Our *Digital Products Newsletter* is the perfect way to stay up-to-date on our latest discounted eBooks, featured mobile apps, and Live Online and On Demand events.

 Learn with real benefits! *HayHouseU.com* is your source for the most innovative online courses from the world's leading personal growth experts. Be the first to know about new online courses and to receive exclusive discounts.

 Enjoy uplifting personal stories, how-to articles, and healing advice, along with videos and empowering quotes, within *Heal Your Life*.

Sign Up Now!

Get inspired, educate yourself, get a complimentary gift, and share the wisdom!

Visit www.hayhouse.com/newsletters to sign up today!

 HAY HOUSE

 HAYHOUSE RADIO
radio for your soul

 HAYHOUSE online learning

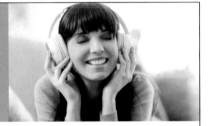

Hay House Podcasts
Bring Fresh, Free Inspiration Each Week!

Hay House proudly offers a selection of life-changing audio content via our most popular podcasts!

Hay House Meditations Podcast

Features your favorite Hay House authors guiding you through meditations designed to help you relax and rejuvenate. Take their words into your soul and cruise through the week!

Dr. Wayne W. Dyer Podcast

Discover the timeless wisdom of Dr. Wayne W. Dyer, world-renowned spiritual teacher and affectionately known as "the father of motivation". Each week brings some of the best selections from the 10-year span of Dr. Dyer's talk show on HayHouseRadio.com.

Hay House World Summit Podcast

Over 1 million people from 217 countries and territories participate in the massive online event known as the Hay House World Summit. This podcast offers weekly mini-lessons from World Summits past as a taste of what you can hear during the annual event, which occurs each May.

Hay House Radio Podcast

Listen to some of the best moments from HayHouseRadio.com, featuring expert authors such as Dr. Christiane Northrup, Anthony William, Caroline Myss, James Van Praagh, and Doreen Virtue discussing topics such as health, self-healing, motivation, spirituality, positive psychology, and personal development.

Hay House Live Podcast

Enjoy a selection of insightful and inspiring lectures from Hay House Live, an exciting event series that features Hay House authors and leading experts in the fields of alternative health, nutrition, intuitive medicine, success, and more! Feel the electricity of our authors engaging with a live audience, and get motivated to live your best life possible!

The Health Habit Hub

**THE PLACE WHERE WOMEN CREATE
THE BEST HEALTH OF THEIR LIVES—
*AND LOVE EVERY MINUTE OF IT.***

Continue your Health Habit journey with Elizabeth and experts from around the world with the 28-Day Kick-Start digital course, new monthly teachings, a comprehensive library of health videos, exclusive e-books, cooking demonstrations, new recipes, wellness inspiration, a supportive community, and more. The Health Habit Hub is available online, 24/7, from anywhere in the world to support your new Health Habit.

> **EXCLUSIVE ENROLLMENT GIFT
> FOR BOOK READERS!**
> Learn more at:
> ElizabethRider.com/membership-gift